All rights reserved by the author.
All contents and corrections are the responsibility
of the author.
Kindle direct 2021

Other work by Beatrice Finn

The value of Hindsight.	1996
Eileen a Mayo girl	2014
Erin Go Braugh	2015
Old Ireland left behind.	2015
Full circle for the Toweys.	2016
The circle of life.	2016
Secrets lies and deceit	2017
Let's be friends	2017
Whispers from Cloontia	2018
Revenge is sweet	2019
Jacintha an Irish Emigrant	2020
Coventry to Indiana.	2020
Jacintha part Three – The Trilogy.	2021
Simply Moira.	2022

Introduction.

Here is some grim but factual information for my great grandchildren, should I ever be blessed enough to have any. If I had the honour of meeting them ahead of me leaving this world, that would be such a bonus for me and I'm sure it would be wonderful for them too.
It may also be of some interest to others who will join this world, long after we have had this experience.
World wars of 1 and 2 in history books they have been written, but maybe not Covid-19 which is effectively world war 3.
Harder however than the previous wars to deal with, as this time it's the invisible enemy staring everyone in the eye and simply waiting for its next vulnerable host.
Whilst watching an Irish scientist on the late late show and holding back her emotions, she shared how if we could see the virus we would not ever go outdoors. Her husband aged 48 years otherwise a fit and healthy man, had just the previous week lost his life to Copvid-19. He of course was one of the statistics of people who had died in Ireland. The United Kingdom lost well in excess of 100,000 people to this dreadful and frightening disease.
The story is and will be written in a poetic and somewhat humorous fashion, as the whole situation unfolds and hopefully one day might come to a satisfactory end.

Beatrice Finn

The very strange year

Of 2020 and 2021

The very awful and invisible enemy named Covid-19
By which not one person was ever
Smitten.
People often had held their own different views
Their opinions they were largely
Written.
Travelling the world to find its very next host
Was all which the virus ever had in
Mind.
Being told that its origin was direct from Wuhan
It sure appeared to be one of a
Kind.

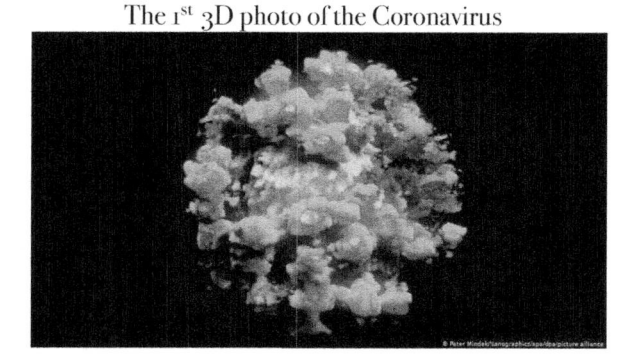

The 1ˢᵗ 3D photo of the Coronavirus

There's so many theories of it to be heard and seen
Some saying that it was started in a
Lab.
Our world scientists overall, they have
Declared
How its origin most likely has come from a bat.
The people of Wuhan in the eyes
Of the world
Can often be so very cruel indeed.
Standing there at their Wet markets'
Should it be wet or dry
Selling animals for many people's greed.

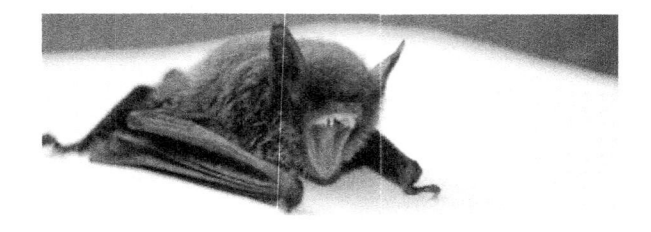

Some dogs some cats and bats being already dead
  Whilst others are slaughtered at the site.
Who would then wish to buy that poor animal
  After having watched it sitting there
        Alive.
From Wuhan the virus travelled very fast indeed
  Killing lots of people standing in its
        Path.
Italy, America and Spain whilst all paying heed
  Didn't know quite how to deal with the
        Aftermath.
As the victim numbers were climbing extremely
        High
  More people were now surely going to die.

Governments everywhere around the whole world
  Were now constantly staying in touch,
Worried that perhaps they were doing too little
  Or for some was it actually all too much.
Very many morgues throughout the whole world
  Had rapidly become overfull and in the
        Heat.
Dead bodies were now sprawled out on some
        Trollies
Which had been lined up in our world's street.

Donald Trump was there still topping the bill
With his many endless and worthless
Tweets.
Telling the American people to drink some
Disinfectant
And how that would keep them up on their feet.
Many people had admired him greatly whilst
Others felt how it may be good if he
Was obsolete.

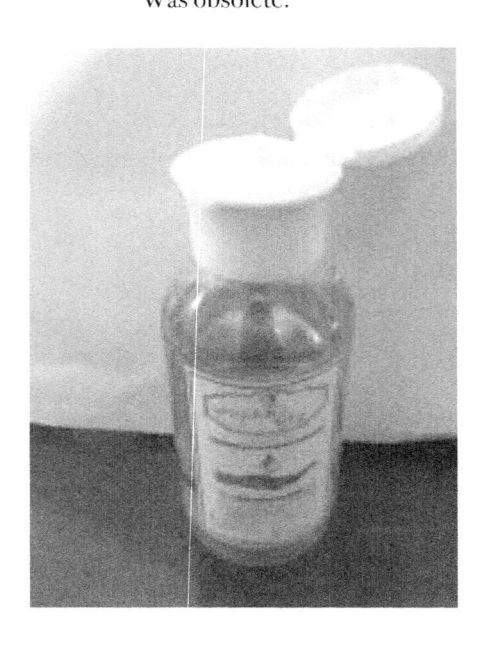

Harsh warnings then came to us from Spain and
Italy
Pointing out exactly what we had lying
In Store.
From our badly effected families living out abroad
Who might never again come to see
Our shores.

Boris stood there almost daily upon his podium
Flanked by his great two men of science
Both he and they were constantly telling us
Amongst many other weird things.
Wash your hands and keep some two
Metres apart
That way we are all then going to save lives.

Protect the precious NHS and everything will be all
Right
Don't worry I've built three more new hospitals
Two which are called Gail and one other is
Called night.
Boris refused to put the country into lockdown
Until that absolutely awful painful night
And then it hit.

Our health secretary Matt Hancock at the opening of one of the new hospitals.

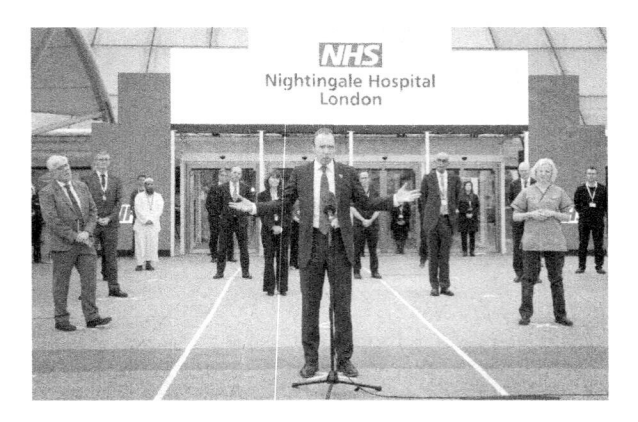

Corona virus eventually had found its host in our
Country
It crossed borders from places very far away
It wasn't fussy who it attacked.
Boris Johnson was one of the many people on
Whose body it did stay.

Boris spent time in St Thomas hospital in London in
Their wonderful department of ICU
Were they the prompts which Boris had then needed
To force his hand for that which he knew
That he should do.
Charlie whilst patiently waiting to take up his seat at
The throne
He did catch the Corona virus too.

The two most protected men in this country
Of their honesty and integrity about their illness
Many people were not too sure.
Then came the government advice we all required
Stay at home, work from home when you can.
Schools were closed, shops were shut, our towns and
Our cities were dead
The country was looking quite forlorn.

Our NHS workers they did go to their place of
Work
Boris said he would do all he could to give them
Perks
Thursday nights he stood outside of
Number 10 Downing Street
It had become a time to clap for our NHS,
Wouldn't it have been better had he given
Them a
More than well-deserved pay rise.
To the very dreaded Covid so many of them did
lose their lives.

This would have helped them feel Respected, perhaps a bit more than doorstep clapping, however with that Boris did not at the time agree.

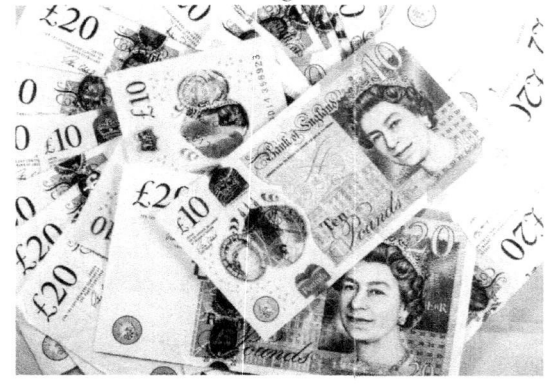

Schools had remained closed for five long months
Children
Were duly kept at home and schooled,
Except the children of our key workers who
Had been
Excluded from the stay at home rules

Examinations for our 16- and 18-year olds
Were
Not allowed to be pursued,
Buckets would surely have been filled by the
Very
Volume of their many tears,
For them being denied of attempting to
Show
What they had learned over the years.

August very soon came around it was now time for
The
Nations exam results to be released.
Seeing how the government bungled all of that
Up
Filled many more buckets with their tears
Nicola Sturgeon put her foot down for
Scotland,
The government would now have to sort it all out.

Boris then decided that he would follow suit
That of course was better news
For the countries students who had by now
Studied for their A levels and their
GCSEs.
On return back to Secondary school their world
Was looking very different there.
Wearing a face mask in all communal areas
Always having to sit on the very same chair.
Mixed in a bubble with their own year
Group only
Heaven forbid that anything
They might share.

Should one group member show any sign of
Covid
The whole year group would get sent home
With instructions of what work to do for
The week
And told to self-isolate for 14 days.
Not fair to our year 11 students who have already
Experienced a very raw deal.
Four months of year ten teaching already
Been missed
How to prepare for next year's GCSEs
Our streets and roads they were largely devoid of
Transport and of people walking near

Being allowed to go outdoors just once daily only
Staying local for exercise people certainly
Saved the pound.
Crazy people had turned very greedy indeed
Hoarding stuff from supermarket shelves
This had occurred well ahead of our lockdown.
They were thinking only of themselves.
Toilet paper had disappeared for weeks on end
Rational people full of frustration with this
Were slowly going around the bend.

Hospital appointments were now very often cancelled
It was tough if whilst waiting you should die
World   health scientists we have now been told
Kept on changing their minds.
About the many different ways to deal with this
Corona virus
In the aftermath of what it left behind.
People died within their nursing homes and in
Many of the residential ones too
Mostly quite elderly and the very highly vulnerable
Raising the death numbers up quite a few
However, some healthy young people they did die too.

For days, then weeks and then months on end
Boris stood talking to the nation
Again, whilst flanked by his top scientists they
Gave the country an explanation.

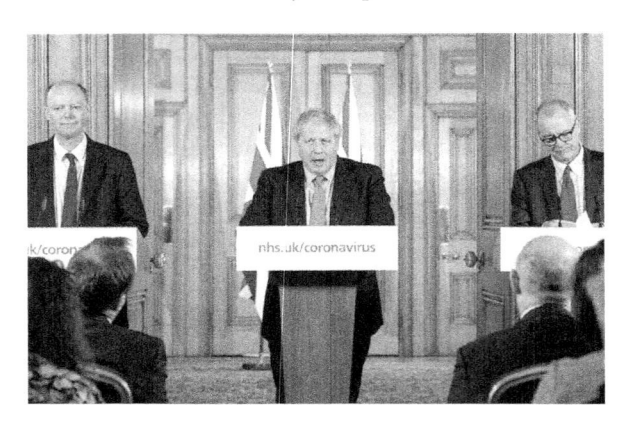

People can no longer mix within each other's
Homes
For many more months to come
To wash our hands and be sure to wear a mask
Has become our regular daily task.
Wearing a mask in enclosed spaces is something
Which we have all already done.

Dominic Cummings held a position of importance
Within our government
It was that of chief adviser to Boris Johnson.
That position for Dominic was quite prestigious and
In our government he felt so high.
Through the very strictest period of lockdown
He proved himself to be quite sly.
Taking a two-hundred-and-sixty-mile round trip
Then defending with his reply.
Johnson received many very unsuccessful appeals
Asking him to give Cummings his permanent leave.

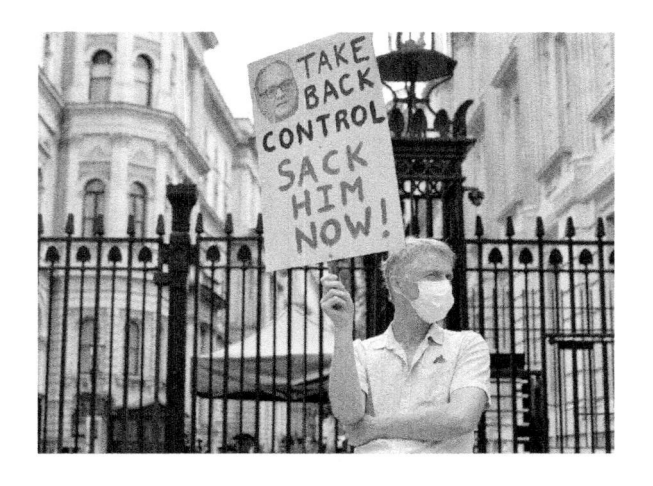

Weddings and such like events were all cancelled
With extremely short notice indeed.
The world had quite suddenly changed beyond
Our recognition and our belief.
Attending your loved one's funeral held some levels
Of restrictions to a person count of ten.
Watching livestream on the internet gave you the
Only possible chance to be with them.
Having to face the other way from each other if from
Different households you did attend.
Oh, what would our ancestors have to say to all of
This.

Then came that day in June which the whole of the
Country was waiting for to hear.
When our lockdown rules could and would
Eventually be released.
Covid-19 otherwise known as 'The Corona Virus
Had quite rapidly brought our country
To its knees.
Change to our rules of freedom were granted for
Almost everyone with many rules being eased.

The still very highly dangerous situation for the
Extremely vulnerable
Boris Johnson was still telling them please.
Don't go out just yet still stay indoors maybe next
Review we will set you all some chores.
Boris set up quite a strong government initiative
For the housebound
Providing them a team of volunteers.

Trying to visit or see your doctor was an impossibility
Didn't happen even if you offered to them a
Substantial fee.
Diagnosis of your illness occurred over the phone
Still tough if you were sitting there ill and
At home all alone.
Nine months or thereabouts later down the line
That situation still hasn't changed.
Is this how our future looks? Will we all survive?
Or will we simply rot at
Home and die?

Consultation with your own hospital specialist
Took place usually through a video link
Imagine how that would not work for deaf people
What on earth would they think?

Some younger generations seemed not to take the
Situation too seriously at all.
Taking part in national and world protests
They at times gathered in big numbers at the mall.
Defying Boris and all which he had said and done
And preached.
Social distancing hand washing and the wearing of
A mask
Was not going to happen at all.

Police officers masked up but not the protesters. Many
police officers were seriously injured at this protest.

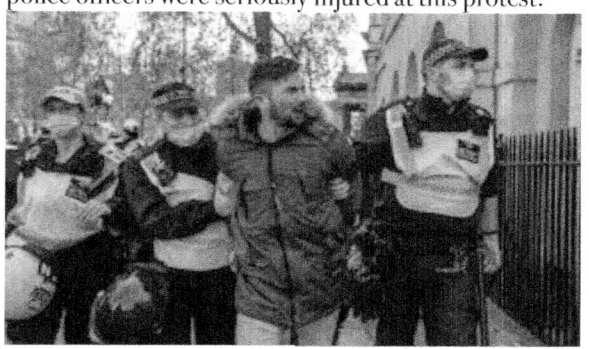

Schools which had returned with some hope were
Sending their year groups home within the
First week.
Telling them to self-isolate for 14 days it would be
Home schooling again with a tweek.
The R number climbed up high again in mid-August
Especially here in Leicestershire
And various other places throughout the country too
Filling people with further fear.

Boris put his foot down putting Leicester back in lockdown
Any breaking of the rules would be given a severe Penalty with a frown.
No one was allowed into another person's house.
Meeting up with friends in their back garden
Was now forbidden too
Even for just a catch up and a cup of tea.

There would be as always had been, some very rare Exceptions
To that very painful rule for the nation.
In order to support the most vulnerable you could Still go inside their home.
Whilst being sure that you always did that with Some very great care
And caution.

Whilst different parts of the country were now put
On those strong and tough restrictions.
Science labs throughout the whole world worked
Tirelessly day and night.
They were on one very ambitious mission
Securing a Covid vaccine
Was now well in their sight.

In the meantime, Boris from his podium talked to
The country once more.
Setting out some further new boundaries causing
Little other than uproar.
Different countries within the United Kingdom
Were definitely not in unison.
Why did Scotland, Wales, Ireland and England
All have their different rules?
What were we to believe and what
Were we all to think?

Was this Covid-19 smart just like our phones?
Finding its hosts in many different ways.
Dependant on where you lived on the night
Or was it a case of the country's leaders being
Obnoxious?
With the thought that only they
Could get this right.

The President of America Donald Trump had
Continued throughout.
With his very many absurd nonsensical tweets and
Refusing to wear a mask.
Despite science proving to us that positive testing
Was well on the increase.
He would stand there on his podium daily
Flanked by his next in line.
Telling the people of the United states of America
Take off your masks this is all going to be fine.

Then came the very sad news which the world was
Certainly not shocked to hear.
It was the beginning of October in this very same
And awful year.
Donald Trump with his wife and first lady had taken
With some others a helicopter flight
Being in very close proximity to each other
And all remaining maskless.
Donald and his wife met their sore plight, The
President and his wife.
Have now both tested positive
For the extremely dangerous Coronavirus.

On October the 3rd in the year 2020 the world was
Given some more sad news.
Donald Trump had overnight been taken into a
Military hospital with Covid-19 or was it
Actually, a ruse?
He allegedly had a raised temperature with lethargy
And goodness knows what else.

Telling the world that age related he is 74 and
Being male,
All combined with his obesity.
Had now somewhat put him in the danger line.
People of the world were now asking if Donald
Might be taking his own advice.
Swallowing
Some Hydroxychloroquine?

Large studies had already shown that this drug was
ineffective as a Covid-19 treatment.

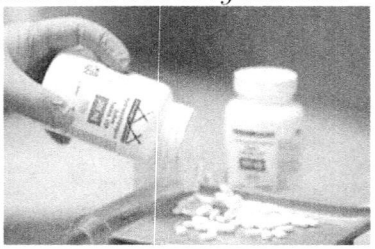

On October the 4th Donald Trump had allegedly
Been given some oxygen to try.
Combined with a highly experimental new drug
Was he going to live or would he die?
The very next day he was behaving like a person
Who was feeling rather smug.

Talking via video link to the nation he told them
How for them he had a great surprise.
He would soon be going outside to greet them
To give them all a spirit rise.
Against the advice of his own top Physicians he then
Organised some cars.
Directly against the quarantine rules Donald left
The hospital to travel afar.

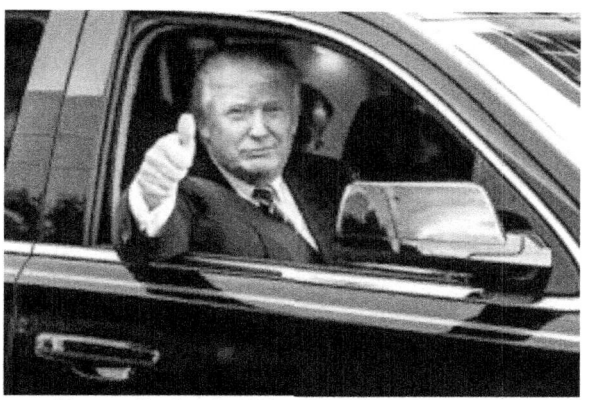

Very sadly for the driver who had no other option
But to drive.
He will be so very lucky if his life he does survive.
Donald's physician quickly told the nation
That the President's behaviour was insane.
That's something most of us have actually known
Since the day he took the reins.

November the 2nd of this year came around very
Fast indeed.
Covid numbers here in England look as though
They are going up with speed.
Boris would have to take some serious action now
He would have to do something at last.
Standing on the podium once more with the two
Scientists by his side.
He told the nation that on the whole once again
That we have to hide.
Our pubs would shut, shops and schools would
Shut, we should work from home when we could.

Go outdoors for essentials only, such as a walk
For exercise.
Do not travel very far away from your home
Put your holiday to one side.
Covid numbers are climbing on the up again
And it's enjoying the ride.
Going back on lockdown for a further four weeks
So many people didn't want to hear.
This would hopefully halt the spread of Covid
But
Would bring our economy to its knees.

On the very eve of the fourth week of our second
Lockdown.
Boris once again addressed the nation
From where he led the country to believe
Was his place of isolation?
Despite him having had Covid earlier on this
Year.
He had shared some close contact to a positive and
Wanted to impress upon the nation.
When your phone app gives you that ping- you
Have to follow the rules and obey.
Don't do like Cummings did, you must self-isolate
For a whole fourteen days.

Talking about Cummings after his very many rows
Within the confines of number 10.
He was eventually instructed by Boris to leave
With immediate effect from then.
That is just what our highly untrustworthy media
Has led the nation to believe.
Cummings having been caught up in a power struggle
With the partner of Boris J.
Apparently brought the whole situation to a head
Which in turn has led to Cummings.
Being given the permanent message of you
Must not stay.

Here he is on his way out and not before time.

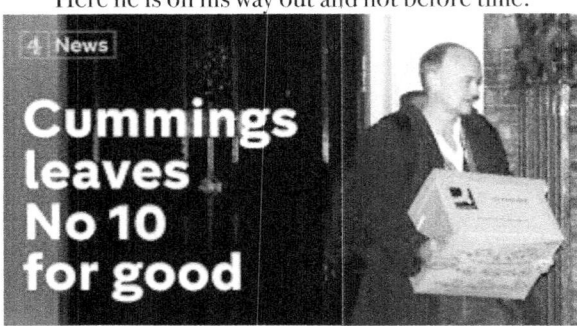

Cummings leaves No 10 for good

Now the four-week lockdown has gone by quite fast
And is almost at its end.
Take a blink and you'll see that Christmas is just
Around the calendar bend.
As the nation waits to see what changes in the rules
We might see.
To our horror and disbelief, the rules of people
Contact have been disagreed.
From the seeing no one indoors to being allowed to
Meet with households up to three.
For a period of six days over the whole of the
Christmas time.
Then we all have to wait and see.

Early in December this year on the second to be
Precise.
Boris stood there on his podium again
Flanked by his very knowledgeable
Men of science.
We as a nation were given the very exciting news
Coronavirus vaccine had been on
This day approved
For its very widespread use.
Having been passed by the regulators gave people
Great confidence
Despite the fact that vaccines generally takes
Some years to present.

So, here's my modest estimation of how this is going
To pan out
Three households mixing together indoors the law
They're going to flout.
Human nature being as it is and now with Boris
Johnsons consent
Nothing's going to hold some people back
On their behaviour some of our lives will depend.

Christmas time comes around but once a year
Of that fact we are all aware
If this virus is not contained, another Christmas
Some of us will never share.
Our country is down on its knee's economy has
Never been so bad
Seeing how very selfishly some people behave
Only serves to make me mad.

Now the vaccine rollout has begun why can't some
People see.
That if only they were less selfish and put Xmas on
Hold
Instead of spouting their innermost thoughts of
I haven't seen my family.
We might all live a bit longer and build a much
Stronger economy.

For what I can see ahead of us Boris has to take some
Responsibility.
He's the one who made the non-sensible six-day
Get together rule.
Couldn't he see that this country is absolutely full
Of fools.
Who wouldn't really care about breaking all of the
Rules.

Saturday the 19th day of December quite late on in
The afternoon.
Boris again talked to the nation from his podium.
Flanked once again by his two scientists one either
Side of him
It was not a moment too soon.
Sharing news about the new Covid virus variant
And how its spreading like wildfire.
Members of the British media at Boris they did rant, as
Once again, he is changing the Xmas plans.

Parts of England where the R numbers are quite high
And still rising.
Are all being placed under what Boris now calls
Tier Four.
With some exceptions if your living in those areas
You can meet with just one person only
It cannot be indoors.
Due to the rapidly rising Covid numbers in all of
Tier four.
There's to be no travelling to other tiered areas, you
Must stay behind your own front door.

If your area has the current status of tiers one or
Two or three.
The previously said six-day rule of seeing family
Meeting up with three households indoors
With no restriction on how many people
Has now been reduced to two
And for one day only.
Boris has told the nation he will in time review
The rules
Some people are left feeling quite confused.

On the 30th of December he will talk to England again
An awful lot can happen between now and then.
Now it's the morning right after the night before
Once again, the nation has been in Uproar.
Media pictures and videos show us this morning
How London trains were last evening
Crammed like tins of Sardines.

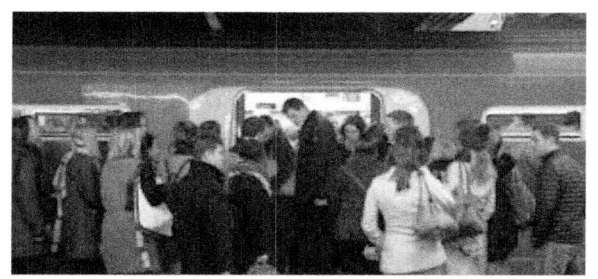

Wanting to escape from the capital ahead of the new
Rules.
With no social distancing or regard for others.
Many had made their minds up to do
As they choose.
When oh when will Boris get to see and to agree
That so many people of this nation
Cannot take responsibility.

Surely, he now needs to make the rules mandatory
Give much more funding to our law enforcers
Get more police presence on our streets.
Will that ever happen under Boris now remains to be
Seen.
After nine months of living with Covid -19 large
Volumes of society have shown.
That in their thinking around the virus rules
They're sense of responsibility has surely not grown.

Oh lord will we ever get back to some degree of
Normality.
This new and alien way of living is the same for
Everyone.
To the exclusion of the highly vulnerable of which
I am one
Being 71 years of age since August yet I comply by
Doing my bit for society before I should die.

Waking up to the world on December 21st I thank our
God that I am still alive
. Then reading some good news on the internet
It now feels like more people will survive
Several countries around the world have now
Barred from England all of their flights
This action seems to have been more than enough
To open up Boris Johnsons eyes.
His rule for tier four has now changed from
Please don't leave
To it now becoming absolutely mandatory.
Dare you to break the rules and you will now see
At your front door
At least one police officer maybe more.

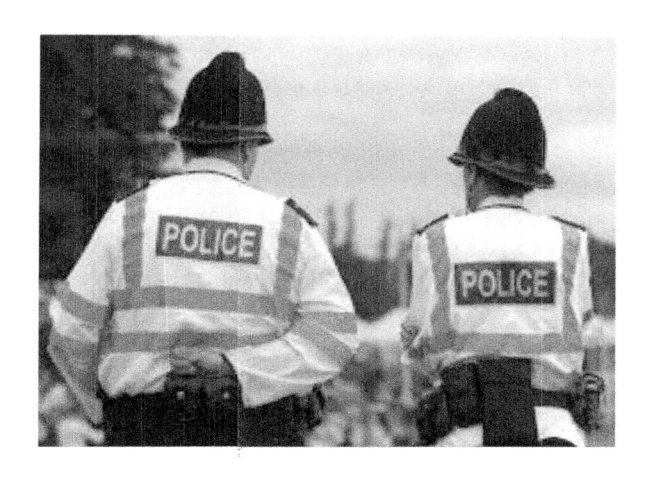

Extra police officers will be deployed to London's
Busy railway lines
Checks will be made on some people's actions
And their behaviour too.
In an attempt to have them tow the Line
Families trying to get out of the capital by car
Will be intercepted.
That hopefully then might bring a sense of
Shame to them
As they will be left feeling quite dejected.

Wednesday 23rd December the nation was once
Again spoken to
This time by our health secretary Mr Hancock
Who informed us that
A 2nd more serious new strain of Covid 19 has been
Detected in Africa
Anyone returning back from there within the next
Few weeks
Will have to immediately go into quarantine.

Wednesday 30th of December and still in the year of
2020
Downing street have now done as they had promised
And completed their review
We all sat with baited breath waiting to hear of
Something new.
Some great news was the first thing to be shared that
The oxford vaccine has now been approved
Millions of doses have been ordered and paid for, so,
We must now wait our turn to be scheduled.

Then from Matt Hancock came the doom and the
Gloom
Due to positive numbers being on the increase
Most of the country is now in new tiers.
For every one, as we are here in
Leicestershire.
Government advice is again to now stay at home
Wash your hands, cover your face and
Give two metres of space.
Oh Lord when will all of this come to an end or will we
Slowly be driven around the bend.

Latest updates are now telling us more bad news
In relation to this new Covid strain
Children are apparently filling up our hospital wards
Is now the latest claim.
On the evening of January 4th in the year of 2021
Boris once more addressed the nation.
Doing that which he should have already done
Weeks beforehand.
He offered us some very worrying also some
Positive Information.

The whole country has once again gone back on
National lockdown
Just as it was in early March last year
Shops are shut, pubs are shut, schools are shut,
We are all living in fear.
The British economy is something from which the
World
Will most likely now want to steer clear.
I did say there was for us some positive news
Which I shall now reveal
In fairness to our government it's been worthwhile
Waiting to hear.

Boris is doing a lot of bragging these days of how
The United Kingdom leads the world.
Being the first to have the biggest roll out ever in the
History of vaccines
Making promises to the nation
Of some dates for us to consider
Saying   the 4 highest groups of vulnerable people
Will be jabbed within the next 6 weeks
We will see.

Many countries around the world are very seriously
Grappling with their own current plight.
France it feels to me is a bit of a disgrace with the
Sharing out of the vaccine to people's rights.
They have only jabbed five hundred arms to date
The world is watching and wondering
Why France is so late.

Despite me being the very grand young age of 71
Years
I have largely managed to this point to control my
Covid fears.
Taking a young person into my care
When with my own grandchildren a hug
I cannot even share.

Now we are back in lockdown with one person in
Every 50 having Covid in our nation.
My foster childs school are placing heavy pressure
For me to send her in next week for
A three-hour examination.
I have given to them quite a crystal-clear
Explanation
As to why that action won't occur
Still the pressure continues via email and text
Message
Today I decided that there's no point in me further
Trying to reason.

I've taken some advice from my son who works within
Education
His explanation to me was very clear
Don't take it personal mum but spell it out to them just
How you feel
Thanking the childs school for their emails with
The information.
I simply shared how she won't be going
As I am working very hard, for me, from this world
Not to disappear.

Right now, just like so many other people I'm very
Frightened of Covid – 1 9
In the last twenty-four-hour period in England alone
More than one thousand people have died
From this disease
And still I'm getting pressure re my foster child
Attending school
I don't however want to make this story about me.

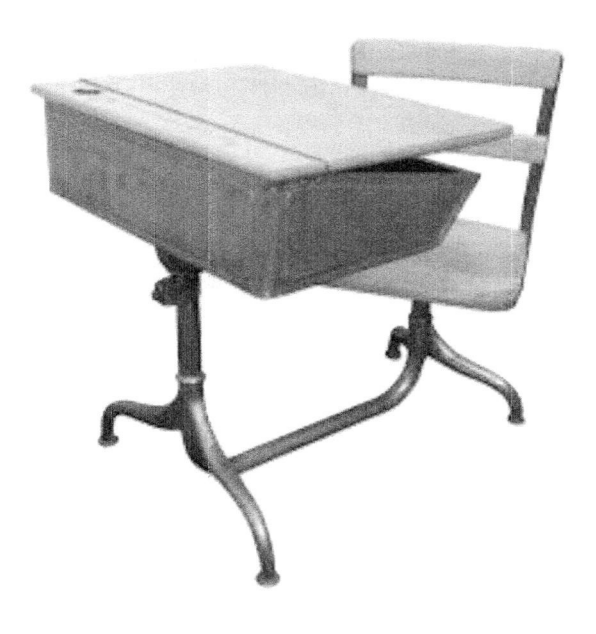

On Monday Jan 4th Matt Hancock once again this
Nation he did address.
Sharing some information
About the biggest vaccine roll out this country
Has ever seen.
Our NHS is now at breaking point with some non
Covid patients
From hospitals being prematurely released.
Being discharged to hotel rooms, where they are
Cared for and well looked after by
A small group of volunteers.
Oh my god it feels as though the country is on its
knees.
I'm very frightened but not for me.

Thinking of the much younger generations and
What their future has in store
Covid-19 Vaccine has to be the way out for
All of us
From this god forsaken mess.
Our police force have had more problems down
In London last weekend
With a head count well in excess of 300 people
A wedding they did attend.
Some people don't seem to understand or to see
Just how very virulent this awful disease
Is and can be.

Today in the headlines came the most despicable
Piece of news
When you'd think that people couldn't stoop or
Go much Lower
We were all reminded just how very low
A low life could really go.
The evidence was right there to stare us in the face.

A small parcel of suspicion to the vaccine making plant
Had been sent
Rendering the unit under evacuation the bomb
Disposal unit in it went
The package was made safe and taken away for
Analysis of its content.

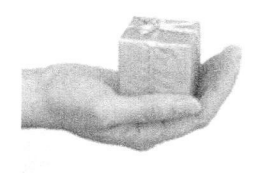

There's some suggestion coming in now from
Germany and some other countries too
That to have the Astra Zeneca vaccine you should
Not be a recycled teen
EU Regulators have however today passed it for
Anyone over the age of 18 years
Saying   that its use is perfectly safe just little
Information on its efficacy
In the older years.
That information has gone some way to
Allaying my deepest fears
We have to take what we are given and for
Me it will be the Astra Zeneca.

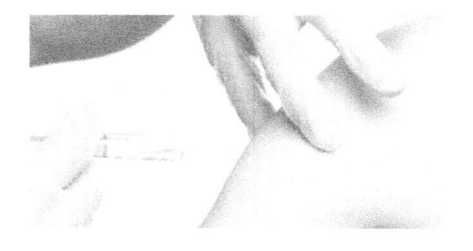

The very 1st day of February in the year 2021
Was a day of great joy and excitement for me
As I have now had my Covid-19 vaccine done
A sore red burning arm was the very end result
I was thinking how this is not like the flu vaccine
And then my overriding thoughts were how
    Covid-19 is simply not like the flu.

The week went forward and I really felt quite sick
    My arm thought it had been hit
    With something like a heavy brick
Being energy depleted meant no walks for me
Aches and pains all over yet nothing to see
Except my poor arm which now looked so thick
    The swelling was there as was the lump
The weekend arrived I felt free from all pain
    A very long walk I then took in the rain.

The country or perhaps the whole world in truth
Knew of a gentleman called
Captain Tom Moore.
Tom was an ex forces man now aged ninety-nine
Who was hoping to give the country a boost
During this awful Covid time
Tom made the decision that he would raise some
Funds
For our struggling health service
He did do the rounds.

He walked with his Zimmer frame around the large
Gardens of his home.
Toms target was to raise at least £1000
Ahead of him reaching his 100th
Year on this ground.
Reality was that the good people of this
Country got behind him
And then Tom walked day upon day.

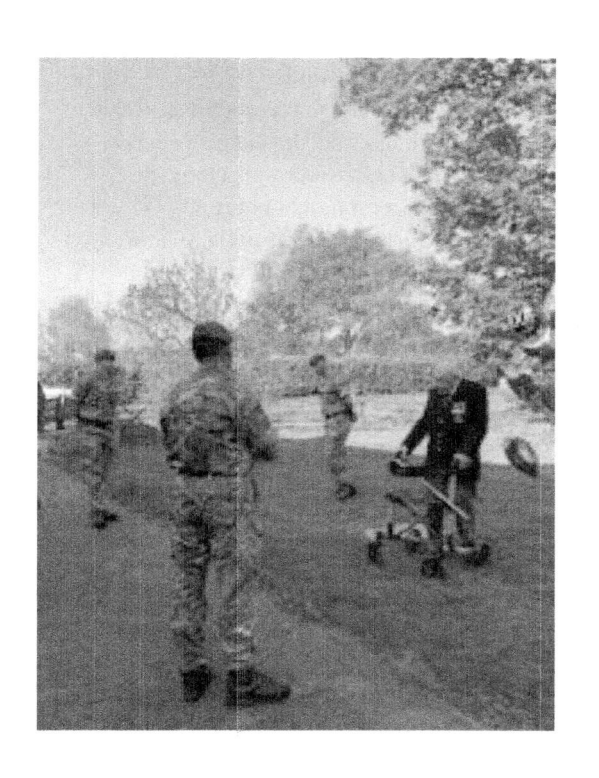

Eventually giving up slightly before his 100th
Year on this earth.
Captain Tom had raised in excess of thirty-two
Million pounds.
His next huge achievement was singing a duet
Together with Michael Ball he did his very best
Their song 'you'll never walk alone' hit
Our charts at number one.
In recognition of Toms efforts in the year of 2020
He was knighted by our Queen.
Later that year Tom decided to take a foreign trip
It would be to the great Caribbean
To spend some badly needed time with his family.

On his return back to England Tom then became
Quite unwell
Suffering from Pneumonia it was easy to tell
A trip to Bedford hospital was something
Which he would need
Then him testing positive for the dreaded.
Covid -19
Was something which he did not deserve.

On the 2nd day of February in the year 2021,
Covid=19
Took Toms life away from his family
No longer would he walk or run.
Being a man of some inspiration, he left a clear
Message for our nation.
The country, the world, had often heard him say
When I have gone keep up with
Your inspiration
Thing 's will one day get better tomorrow is a new
Day.

Tributes have poured in for Tom from around the
Whole of the world
Sir Captain Tom is now a man who will never
Never be forgotten.
For the way in which he stood for the spirit of
Optimism
Boris Johnson has sent out a national
Request.
That to honour this noble gentleman
Tonight at 6pm
We should all follow his address.
By doing a clap for Sir Tom Just like we all did
Last year for the NHS.

Covid variants and new strains are now becoming
Quite prevalent
People arriving at English Borders from certain
Red list countries
Will now go into quarantine.
This boundary is now mandatory for all
Attempt to break it and you
Won't have much fun at all.
More information regarding this is soon to be
Released.

More updates on what's coming next from our Health
Secretary Matt Hancock
Anyone entering the United Kingdom from now
Has a quarantine fee of £ 1700 to pay
Should they lie or try to hide details of where they've
Travelled from.
Behind prison gates for ten years is where they will
Have to stay.

Some back benchers are in uproar saying how the
Punishment is too severe
Matt Hancock is sticking to his guns telling them
This is the biggest threat to public Health
That any of us alive today have ever seen
So yes, the prison deterrent it will stay
And will be executed
Should there be a need.

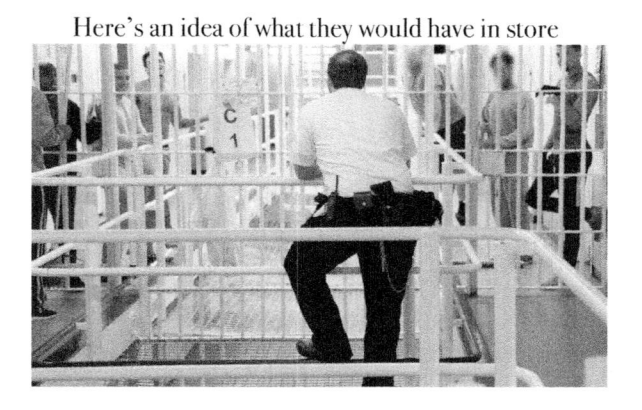

Here's an idea of what they would have in store

February 15th and Boris spoke to the nation
Once again
Feeling very proud of how many people
Have now had the vaccine
So many questions to him were put
From reporters wanting to know how and when
Will we get out of this awful rut?

Of his handling of this whole Covid situation
Some people say
Boris has made a terrible mess
Perhaps to some degree he has
However, asking him if he can guarantee there will
Be no further lockdown.
Seemed an impossible question to answer and to
My brow brought a frown

Waking up to the news on this Tuesday morning
There's lots of suggestions and giving us
All some warning
That this awful virus is mutating once again
Will this for us mean a further lockdown
Or will the fight we actually win.
Our world health organisation have been in Wuhan
For quite some time now
Their purpose there is an attempt to establish if and
How
That's where Covid-19s life it did begin.

This is how our scientists; our hospital doctors and nurses have to dress, when working on the front line with their Covid patients.

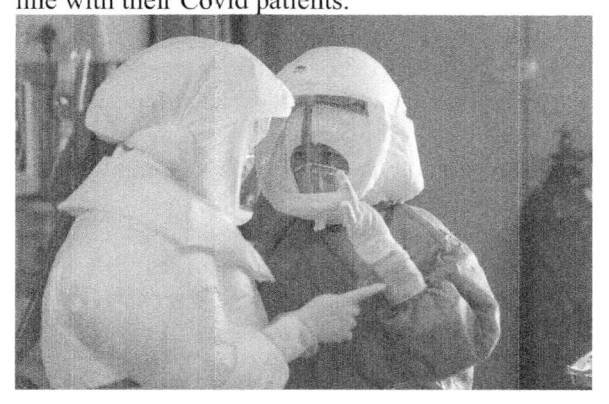

Information coming to us from professor Watson
Has the strong suggestion that
The onus is not on just Wuhan
Scientists of the world now need to look
Outside of Chinas borders as well as within
The man feels that Covid-19 probably started from
A water source
In which it was transferred from animal to human
Also in his summing up to date
Professor Watson did conclude
The possibility of the virus having escaped from a
Laboratory in Wuhan
Is not out ruled.

Monday February the 22nd and here we are again
With Boris standing up there on the podium
Flanked by the same two science men.
He has given the country some dates where things
Will begin to change
Keeping it all within a reasonable range.
Our schools being the 1st to open on March the 8th
Its looking as though life is getting back
To some form of normality
Before its too late for me.

Boris and his scientists were all now very clear, that
Normality as we once knew it
Is now quite near
He's hoping to never have to go back to lockdown
Again.
The vaccine will protect us from within
Despite the very many people
Who from this awful virus they have lost their lives
Many of this country's population
On the Covid-19 vaccine they will not agree to rely.

The strong message now coming from Downing Street.
Is that with our families we will soon be able to Meet.
The vaccine refusers may submit to persuasion
As the government considers
A Covid passport for the whole nation.
Conspiracy theorists they would and do Complain.
It's a chip going under our skin
Which would drive us all insane.

Its February the 25th and here we are once again.
This time its Gavin Williamson
Our education secretary
With a health scientist up there on the podium
Telling the nation of governments how new plans
That to see our children educated
Is the country's demands.

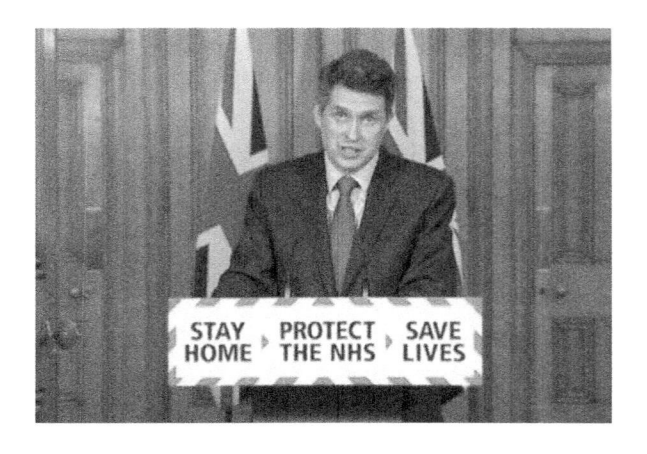

Extending on the school year by a few weeks or more
His plan is to give our teaching staff many more chores
To make this successful government are doing
. Their part
By throwing more money into the education pot.
With the strong hopes of a better future for our nation.

Three hundred and two million pounds extra cash to
Allow all of our children to catch up.
With two hundred million extra for secondary
School pupils
In the hopes that their exam results will then reflect
Their hard work.
How to grade our students this year has been quite a
Challenge to say the least.

With months of missed learning spent at home
To follow the students wish this government has
At last agreed
That they will trust our teacher's judgement with a
Robust system for appeal.

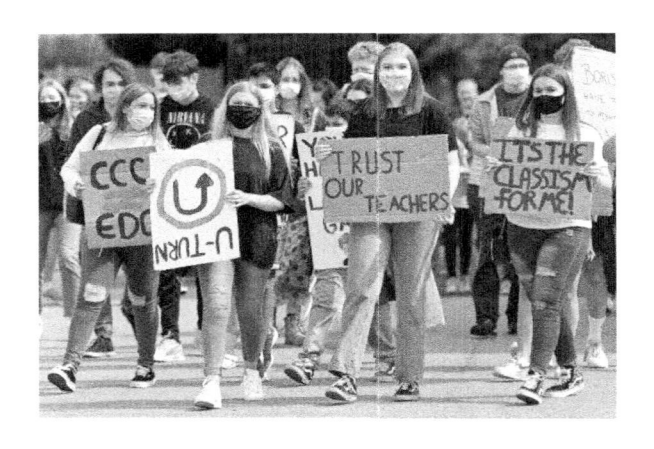

Despite all which Boris has said about our exit from
Lockdown.
And how as we go through the stages all leading up
To June.
One of those stages which will be that we can
See our family
Was saddened and almost feels like it's in ruin.

Disappointing information came out to the nation
Telling families how we should all hold fire
Children should not be hugging their
Grandparents, even if they've had the vaccine
That hugging should be avoided until we are
Absolutely sure of the effectiveness at this time.

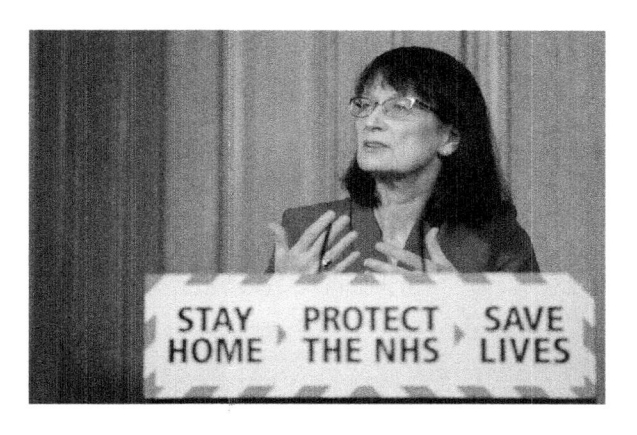

Hearing that information from doctor Jenny Harries
In her role as England's deputy chief medical officer
Whilst it might have brought to our eyes
Some more tears
Our commitment we have to give to her.

It's now Friday February 26th and here we are again
Update was led by Matt Hancock and his scientific men
With input from Professor Jonathan Van Tam
Matt Hancock shared about the numbers
And how they are coming down.
Professor Van Tam was not at all subtle
As he told us we have to keep our feet on the ground.

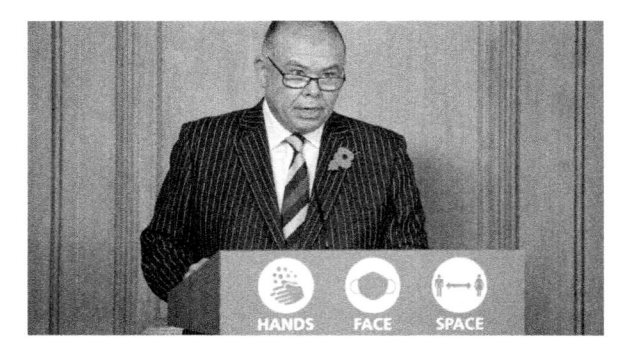

Sharing also with the nation how his email inbox is on Overflow
From people saying I've had the vaccine, so to see Family and friends can I now go? Well NO.
It feels almost embarrassing belonging to a nation Which would exercise that level of stupidity.
That after all the many times we have now been told
They still need to ask the basic question of are we free?

With good continuity of his knowledge and his advice
He once again told the nation which behaviour is
Wrong
And which behaviour is right
Professor Van Tam he was clear with his sternly
Spoken words
As a very sobering warning he did give to the nation
Weathers warmer weekends upon us
Don't think Covid's all over, we still have to stay at
Home and obey.
Everyone should remain to be disciplined
Hang on just a few more months.

Van Tam was stern in his briefing that lockdown in
Essence will end in June.
However, if certain areas continue to break the
Rules.
With data showing us the R is going up, to put those
Areas back in Tiered lockdowns.
The government will not hesitate.

Friday the 5th of March and Matt Hancock has spoken
To us again.
Sharing information which confirms everything is
Looking less grim.
The vaccine rollout is well on target
And doing its job very well.
Soon we should all feel some release
From a year which has felt like something from hell.

Scientists having travelled to Wuhan in January of
This year.
Spending time on their investigation in the hopes to
Allay some fears.
Have now on the 7th of March been told that their
Interim report summarizing their investigation
Has been scrapped.
There will be some further investigations when they
Can find a better source
Not be dependant on what the government of China
Tells to them.
And what they choose to share.

In the meantime, amidst this awful world crisis
Many peoples Mental Health has really taken
        A toll.
Prince Harry and his wife Meghan Markle took
        To the air waves.
Despite the awful timing due to Harrys Grandad
        Prince Phillip.
Being in hospital treated for a heart condition
        And he's 99 years of age.
  Their own story was going to be told.

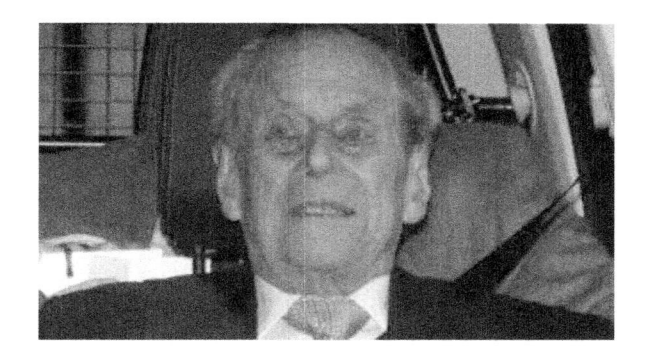

Harry having lost his mother in a car crash in
France
When he was just 12 years of age
His view was that she had been harassed
By the press
This had clearly caused Harry an awful lot of stress.

Harry wanted out!!

In attempts to protect his wife and child from them
Harry and Meghan made their decision
To leave this country and live abroad
Where their media experience
Would hopefully be much less.

Harry with Meghan, Archie and their baby daughter which Megan is carrying.

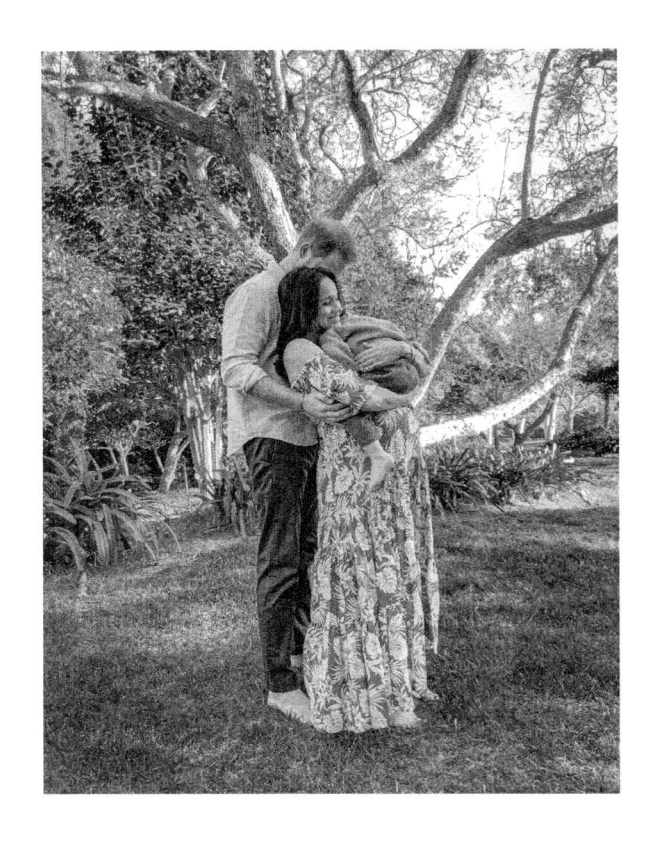

Harry often appears to be living life in his late mothers'
Footsteps.
In their interview to the world - they both spoke of
Their own poor Mental Health.
Harry shared how his father had cut him off.
His brother William had gone down the very same path
Is this really very kind behaviour.
They had both suffered and endured the same wrath.

Diana with William and Harry on one of their many fun days together.

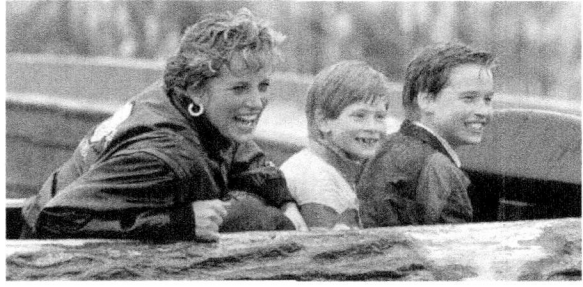

Knowing that William will most likely one day be
King
I ask myself this question.
In the light of his family rift due to his lack of
Understanding for his brother.
Is he really suitable to become our King?
Remaining in a stifled stuck up manner he's more
Like
His father than his mother.
Is he simply staying in solidarity with the monarchy?
Or does he have a genuine
Dislike for his brother.

The answer to that question we will probably never
Know!!!

Here's an admission of my very strong digression
Now I'm back to the topic at hand.
There's some news in the headlines today
Which maybe looks a little bad for the people
Of our land.
The medicines regulator for Austria has suspended
A batch of our own Astra Zeneca Vaccines.
Post some information of some patients developing
Blood clots.
With some more serious and dangerous outcomes
After having their vaccine.

Saturday March 13th has brought us some more
Diverse information.
A gentleman of whom I've never heard of
With the name of Laurence Fox.
Has told the country of his view on the
Idea of holiday passports.
Saying that vaccine should be the same as
Voting.
That it should be a sovereign
Choice.

The actor Laurence Fox

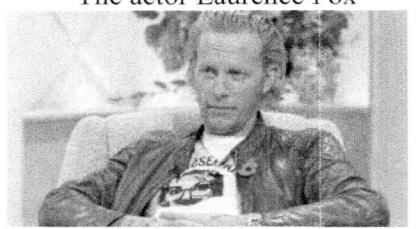

London's chief nurse who is Mr Martin Machray
Had given a speech on that very same day
He told a Westminster webinar.
Of the importance of the vaccine to continue
To be seen as a force of good.

Others in that meeting felt how the words from Mr
Fox.
Regarding deaths registered from Covid-19 to be
False
Were such an insult
To the very many people whose loved ones they
Had lost.

Mr Fox who is an actor and leader of the
Reclaim party.
Said he is going to stand on may 6th to
Become London's Mayor.
That should he be elected to that position
He will ensure that the country is treated fair.
His idea of how to do that is
He will end our lockdown.
In those statements isn't he missing a very
Large point.
The Coronavirus act states that only a Prime
Minister
Can get the country out of lockdown.

Children having now returned back to their
Classrooms.
Was our first step taken out of this country's
Mess.
Being provided twice weekly with rapid flow
Testing kits.
I'm thinking that as a nation
We are all quite impressed.
We are now waiting for the next step out with
Baited breath.

On March 23rd there is going to be a national
Doorstep vigil.
It will be a minute's silence to mark the
Countries
First Covid lockdown.
Prominent buildings throughout the country
Will be lit up.
With a request for doorsteps to follow suit.
In remembrance of all of those who lost their
Lives.
If this will be of much comfort
To their families
I'm not actually too sure.

It's now Wednesday March 17th and yet another
Covid update.
From Professor Van Tam came some news of
Our potential fate.
Reassuring the nation that for a blood clot worry
Worry we should really pay no heed.
The vaccine is definitely what we need.
Making his point to us he read out prospects of
How taking a simple paracetamol can have so
Many side effects.

Now its March 23rd upon us and Boris once
Again has taken to the podium.
This time it was mostly for reflection as it's a
One-year anniversary.
Of the day we first went into lockdown.
Making some acknowledgement
Regarding our government's mistakes.
Of their lack of knowledge of Covid's spread
From and by those who were so often
Asymptomatic.

Looking at the world overall as a whole today
England looks to be doing pretty well.
With a very high percentage of vaccine uptake
It looks as though we're getting out of this hell.
Vaccine refusers working in care homes
May have their choice removed.
In order to protect our old and vulnerable a
Covid vaccine is required.
For the refusers it may become mandatory as
Of their refusal our government is getting tired.

Looking through the media they are at it
Again
On putting their own take on what is not
Much more than a whim.
Stating that children could be vaccinated as
Early as August this year.
Is not necessarily the case says Professor
Adam Finn.

March 30th and here we are again with more
Updates in the news.
World health scientists investigating in
Wuhan.
Have had a leak on their views.
Stating the most likely cause for Covid-19
Has been through bat transmission.
Some of the scientists have shared their own
Decisions.
Regards some content of the reports
Which in part.
Have been written by the government of
Beijing.

It's now Saturday April 3rd the controversy still
Continues.
Several countries are now putting on hold
Our home-grown vaccine
Astra Zeneca.
Others like for example Germany are stating
It's not to be given to anyone under the
Age of 60 years.
All this hype concerning blood clotting is
Accelerating people's fears.

Boris states that it's all political yet a link has
Been made.
Which connects our Astra Zeneca.
To potential blood clotting problems.
In females of a certain age.
We have waited for the top scientists to check
Exactly where we go from here
They're reliable assessment is that
We should all take the vaccine
Without fear.

Its Monday April the 5th and another Covid
Update.
Looking especially at travel arrangements
And how these are mostly going
To be our fate.
All travel abroad will be colour coded
Just like a set of traffic lights.
Boris also told the nation how coming out of
Lockdown
So far is on track and won't be late.

Taking a foreign holiday to all of the green list
Countries.
Will hold some cost extra for everyone.
Even when fully vaccinated we will still
Need to take a private Covid test.
On our return home to England from countries
Which are on the green colour coded list
If the country is on the amber colour coded
List.
We have to take a test and self-isolate at
Home for ten days.
If returning from a red colour coded country
We take a test then quarantine.
At our own very high expense.
In a government chosen hotel for two weeks.

Shops, gyms, hair salons and some pubs will all
Open up next Monday as
Per the original plan.
Personally, I cannot wait to have a hair cut
I'm looking rather like gypsy Anne
Who gypsy Anne is I do not know.
It just popped into my head and works with the
Poetic flow.

Looking further afield world-wide People are
Being treated badly by officials.
A man has died from the punishment given
To him
For breach of their strict Covid curfew in
Indonesia.
Being forced to do 300 squats like exercise
Proved itself to be too much.
His body fitted and then his heart died.
Police there have told his partner that no such
Punishment exists within their force.
There will be an investigation, seeing
The officers dealt with
In due course.

On another serious matter of some very high
Importance indeed.
The world was this day Saturday April 10th
Given some very sad news.
Her majesty Queen Elizabeth told our nation
How her husband Prince Phillip aged Ninety
Nine years.
Had this morning peacefully gone to meet
His maker.
The year of 2020 and the year of 2021.
Will be remembered for a very long
Time to come.

Tributes continue pouring in from so many
Dignitaries around the world.
Today there will be a national death gun
Salute at midday.
Prince Philip will be honoured.
For his life which was a colourful array.
Forty-one-gun shots will be fired at the rate
Of one per minute.
He will not be having a state funeral nor
Will his body lie in state.

Prince Phillip will rest at Windsor Castle until
His funeral date is upon us.
Those were the wishes of the man himself
He wanted a send-off which would be free
From hassle and from fuss.

Back to the Covid -19 issues and the vaccine in
Particular.
I'm feeling very honoured to say that I have
This morning had my second dose.
As a nation we are all so fortunate and so very
Blessed indeed.
To have at our disposal some scientists who are
Some of the world's very best.

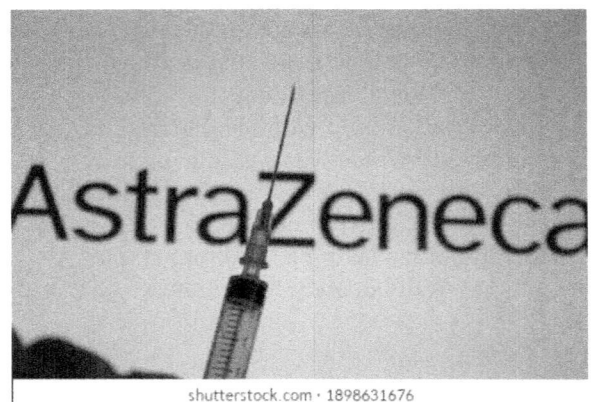

Now we have Tuesday evening April 20th 2021
We've had yet another briefing
From Boris and part of his team.
Tonight, they were joined by a general practice
Doctor member
She is called doctor Nikita Kanani and she works
as a gp in London.
In addition to her role as Medical director
For primary care to NHS
England.

Supporting Boris in all which he said about
Having another line of medical defence
She did a very good job.
An anti-viral task force will be set up
With hopes for a tablet or a simple pill
The idea being that if you
Test positive.
The pill will hopefully prevent you from
Becoming too ill.

Boris has this evening given the nation quite
A stern warning.
That despite the progress made by lockdown
And the super uptake of the vaccine
The last of Covid we have not yet seen.
Our British scientists firmly believe
That there will be a further wave later on
This year.

That Covid is something with which we will
Have to live with
Wear our face coverings, keep our distance.
Testing twice weekly now available to all
What a world our children are adapting to
Covid passports will probably be the next call.

We have to try to find a way to put Covid
Back in the box.
Before the progress we've made
Finds itself getting lost.
Despite the very high vaccine uptake
There are some whom that action
Didn't take.
Perhaps a mandatory Covid passport could
Be what's required.
Should people wish to live a full life.

A front leading scientific member from the
World Health Organisation.
Has this morning given to the world a
Warning.
That we should not become complacent
Saying that in terms of the new variants
There's going to be another deadly
One.
Which will penetrate the vaccines
And how that is a fact of it
Will be when and not if.

We now have Monday morning April the 26th
Checking up with the world news
It shows this virus is still very rampant
In countries where people still run loose.
People living in India
Are rapidly losing their lives.
World news has shown outside of their
Hospitals.
People dying on their stretchers whilst they
Wait to be seen.
Their health system is absolutely
Overwhelmed
With a desperate shortage of oxygen.

The super-rich of India are hiring private jets
Taking themselves to other countries.
Where the virus rampancy is much less.
Some having flown to Great Britain
I feel is very dangerous for us.
Now India has been placed on the red banned
Countries list
I feel for this country but for us it can only be a
Plus.

In America the situation could be better than
It currently is.
More than five million people have rejected
Their 2nd vaccine.
Some saying they have huge concern
Regarding potential side effects.
Whilst others claim to know better than our
World scientists.
Stating a 2nd vaccine is not required
That one is more than enough.

Coronavirus has certainly turned this world
On Its head.
Millions and millions of people due to it
Are now dead.
Some of us tow the line by abiding by the
Covid rules.
Whilst others world-wide go on rampage
Demonstrating their abuse.

Looking at this very poignant picture of our
Queen
Sitting alone at her husband's last goodbyes.
Adhering to all of the Covid rules
I'm sure there were tears in her eyes.
Makes me feel ashamed of the
People.
Who live their lives with no regard?
Going out in large gatherings
Making trouble.
When like the rest of us and our Queen
They should stick to their own bubble.

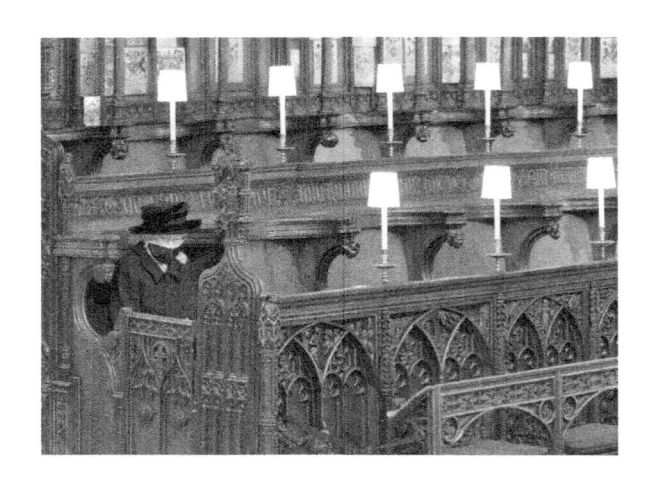

This very weekend which we have just come
Through
Has again seen hundreds
On the streets of London protesting with their
View.
There are people who state that Covid is not
Real.
That the world has created a big conspiracy
Don't they watch the news?
Or follow what's shown by the media.
Whatever must be their view of what's currently
Occurring in India.

It's Wednesday morning and it's now the 28th of
April.
Looking at the news channels
India is still experiencing the most awful fate.
People are still dying on stretchers
In the street.
Hospitals continue to be overwhelmed.
As patients' needs they cannot meet.
Beyond heart-breaking to see.

The world knows it has to send support as
That will be the only way out.
Despite Covid being worldwide, some
Countries now have it in their control.
The United Kingdom has provided to India.
Some badly needed medical gear.
Ventilators and oxygen concentrators.
Will all hopefully reduce their fear.

However the crisis in India continues with
People dying from Covid almost
Every minute.
Hundreds of people are queuing up outside
Of oxygen making plants.
Paying to have their cannisters refilled.
Then take to the hospitals for their loved
Ones
On it whose lives depend.

Men seen here with an oxygen cylinder

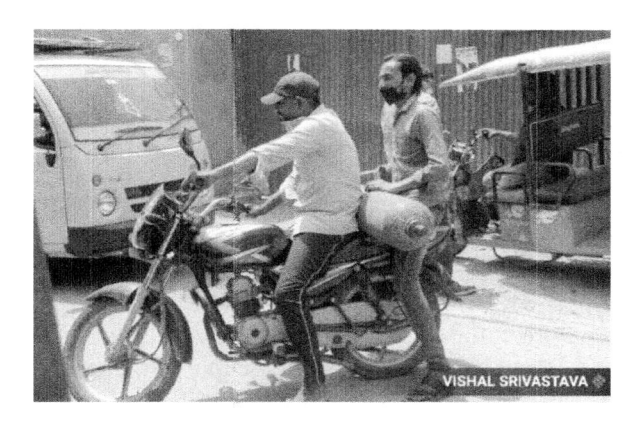

Back to our own United Kingdom situation.
Downing street once again tonight spoke
To the nation.
It was good news all round regarding the
Covid-19 vaccine.
Unexpectedly high rates in reducing Covid
Transmission.
Professor Van Tam is delighted to have seen.

Now it's Friday the 30th of April I'm looking at
The world news.
Israel has been taken out of lockdown
However, the country still has rules.
Last night those rules were badly broken.
When a religious festival people did attend.

Authorisation was set for ten thousand people
More than thirty thousand did attend.
Pushing and shoving created a stampede
Over forty lives came to their end.
All in the name of honouring their god.
Their thinking is hard for me to comprehend.

It's now the weekend of May the 2nd and a
Covid trial we have duly seen.
Legally set up by the government.
Six thousand people they have been.
In attendance at an all-night rave in
Liverpool.
No social distancing or masks required.
Just a negative Covid test before they arrive.

Monday the 3rd of May and I have listened to
Professor Adam Finn.
He has now stated that in Autumn the new
Vaccine will begin.
It will be offered to children at secondary
Schools.
He's hoping the uptake will be more than a
Few.
Repeating what he has previously stated to the
United Kingdom and to the world.
Everyone should take the vaccine
When their time is due.

Reading up on the daily news today was very
Enlightening
When you think that fraudsters can stoop
No lower
The reality feels quite frightening
Scammers targeting people on their doorstep
On the pretext of selling Covid-19 testing kits
Some people are sadly gullible.
That's where the fraudsters made their hits.

Looking further round the world we can clearly
See.
Some good work being implemented by
Jacinda Arden.
She is the government leader for New Zealand.
The lady has from the very beginning held a
No nonsense approach.
Putting the country or parts of it in lockdown.
Immediately cases of Covid had begun to
Show.

Currently the situation in her country is flying
High.
To take the Covid vaccine is mandatory, or to
Your job you may well say goodbye.
The rule of mandatory is applicable to workers
In areas of isolation and facilities of
Quarantine.
Also including government agency workers.
Who are performing border control.
Some people on customs duties have reportedly
Been sacked.
Due to their refusal to take the Covid jab.

From this lady some lessons could very well be
Learned.
For none of the sacked workers compensation
Will not be received.
Their positions will remain open as a matter
Of need.
The sacked workers are now all feeling very
Disgruntled indeed.

With one sacked lady telling a reporter how
For her position.
There was insufficient need for her to have
Had a vaccine.
Why oh why do some people think
That they should be the decision makers.
Of putting other people's lives at risk.
Doesn't the world scientists view
Count for anything to them.

Now we're getting to the point where foreign
Holidays will once more begin.
The rules are set out clearly by Boris.
Depending on which coloured list
Your destination is in.
The green list means no quarantine required
If you're on the amber list.
For at least five days you must hide.
Destination from the red list to our country is
Expensive news.
Requiring everyone to go direct to a
Government chosen quarantine hotel.
That's where people will remain for ten days.
At a cost of £1750 per person which
You the traveller will have to pay.

The dreadful Covid catastrophe which remains
Still rampant in India
Is according to scientists a warning to us all.
He shared how the world needs to adopt a
Global view on vaccines.
Otherwise to India's current Covid situation.
Every country has the potential to fall.

Vaccine minister for the United Kingdom has
This morning given us some very good news.
Stating that Covid-19 will become an endemic
Just like the seasonal flu.
That as our world leading vaccine rollout
Continues.
How we are on course to have crushed the threat
Of
More devastating waves of Covid-19.

After that quite good news then comes the bad.
A government document has been
Leaked.
According to a reporting lad.
Clusters of the Indian variants have now been
Found in the UK.
Update on these case numbers should have
Been disclosed today.
However, as its now local elections time.
Disclosures of this have been postponed for a
While.

According to the Guardian newspaper which is
Held in pretty high esteem.
Leaked internal documents from public health
England show.
That the ongoing risk to public health from
These variant's
Is the very opposite of low.

Forty-eight clusters of the Indian variants have
Been found.
Some in places of religious gatherings and some
In other grounds.
Let's hope Boris and the scientists can turn this
All around.

India in the interim is demonstrating a see no
Evil hear no evil motto.
Where covid-19 death numbers are unseen.
We are now led to believe by their media
That their government.
Incites fear and has them cook the books.
Choosing not to be transparent
Does not give the country a very good look.

Meanwhile back here in England our numbers
Of positive tests are slowly on the incline
Perhaps not too surprising as the country is
Opening up in line.
With government rules and boundaries.

Despite the evidence of this incline, our vaccine
Task force chief Mr Clive Dix.
Has said the virus will no longer be circulating
In Britain by the middle of this summer.
That every adult will have been offered the
Vaccine
That's its uptake will keep Covid on the decline.

Human challenge Covid study trials, are set to
Begin in the United Kingdom.
Volunteers between the ages of eighteen and
Thirty years.
Will be injected with Coronavirus
This virus exposure will occur in a safe and
Controlled manner
As medics and health professionals continue
To monitor their health.

It's now Monday the 10th of May and we've had
Another Downing street update.
Boris and his scientists talked us through
What's on our plate.
Appealing to everyone to still do the right
Thing.
He shared about how the country will be
Opening up once again.

On Monday the 17th of May this country will
See many changes.
Travel restrictions will no longer be in place
Dining out indoors having friends and family
Come to stay.
All will come into place should the data remain
The same.
Telling the nation that we are on track for a full
Lock down lift.
On the 21st of June if there aren't any rifts.

His advice to everyone as from that date going
Forward.
Is that we should be back to what we knew as
Normal.
But should still exercise caution and some
Common sense.
Speaking of the new Covid variants and their
Resistance to our Vaccine.
He confirmed that the Indian one is a global
Concern.
Due to its ability of transmissibility
How that will all work out we will need to wait
And see.

It's now Wednesday morning on the 12th day
Of May.
Scientists throughout the country are trying
To have their say.
What's written in the media if we are to
Believe.
A third wave of Covid will be on its way.
Pre-empted by the Indian variant.
Which looks as though it's not going to go
Away.

Telling Boris that he should not open up in
June
That if he does then the nation's health will
Once again go to ruin
Not only have the scientists stated that many
More deaths will be seen
Grimly their predictions are that it will be some
People
Who have received their vaccine.

Here we are again on Thursday morning of
May the 13th
Scientists continue to warn Boris Johnson
About the Indian Variant.
Their suggestions being that if he doesn't
Take more control.
This country will fast become like India losing
People by the score.
Just what he will do we will have to wait and
See.

Some good news for the people of England this
Morning in relation to our gps
Since the onset of Corona virus.
Our doctor we have not been able to see.
The system of telephone triage
Is how the last year and more has been.
Our NHS England has now looked again at
Advice which has been formalised by them.
As of today, the rules have changed.
Where every person who requests face to face
A doctor they will now be able to see.
Telephone consultation should remain if
That should be a patient's request.
Decision will then be made by the doctor.
Regarding what they think is best.

Now Friday the 14th of May and Boris talked
To us again.
Together with one of his scientific men
Stating we must be very sensible and not act
On a whim.
Further easing of restrictions will go ahead as
Planned.
Keeping a close eye on the Indian variant and
How it spreads throughout this land.

Some people in this country have behaved very
Badly indeed.
Putting others at risk fuelled by their greed
Greed isn't always for a monetary gain
People have demonstrated that fact by their
Recklessness in the main.
Shown through large gatherings with no respect
For those who lost loved ones to Covid and
Are in pain.

The new Indian variant is now spreading like
Wildfire
Especially in places like Blackburn, Bolton
And the north East.
Thousands extra doses of the vaccine have
Been deployed to those areas
Will we see the required uptake remains to
Be seen.

Accepting that the new travel rules are in our
Favour.
For border control at airports
It's a time-consuming labour.
Having to manually check every passengers
Details concerning Covid

Requests are going into government from some
Airport bosses who are feeling.
Very overloaded.
Pointing out that there has to be a better way
Before staff take time off feeling ill.
Bosses have suggested to Boris
That the whole process becomes digital.

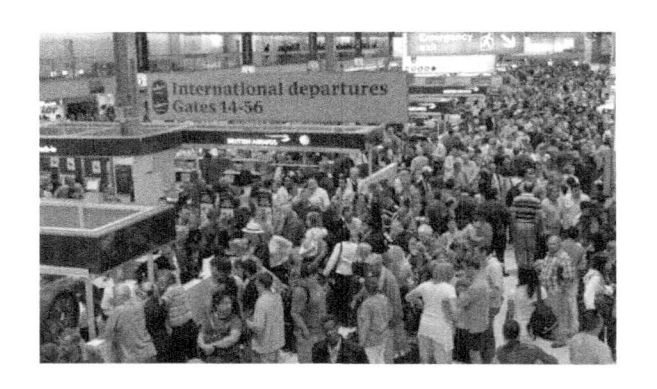

Some have suggested that queuing time is
Taking longer than many flights.
Few are wearing masks
Social distancing is not applied.
When oh when will people ever see.
That they can be and often are
The cause of spreading this just like a flea.

In terms of the anti Covid rules mobs, they
Have now taken it a step further.
Gathering outside of vaccination centres
For the purpose of vaccine prevention.
My thoughts are similar to how they were
Last year.
Bring in the British army that would soon
Get them off the streets.

Tonight, we have listened to Matt Hancock our
Health secretary.
He shared how now there's many people
Back in hospital with Covid-19.
Right across the age range with some in
Intensive care.
Every single patient who's now in that situation.
Has previously been offered a vaccine but for
Whatever reason.
They declined for their arm with the needle to
Share.

Government have been looking at Bolton with
The vaccine rollout.
Where the new Indian variant has doubled
It's numbers.
Over the past few days.
Young people as young as eighteen years of
Age.
Have now made their attempts by getting in line
Only to be refused.
Boris is sticking to the priority list. People
Will have to wait.

I can only imagine and can only take a small
Guess.
That the people of Bolton and the north East
Are now living with regret.
Its been that refusal to follow all the rules
That will probably put Bolton back under
Economic duress.
Government and our scientists have with us
Been consistently transparent.
That following the safety rules combined with
Accepting the vaccine.
Will always be our only way out of this awful
And very deep ravine.

The world of awful conspiracies continues to be
Stimulated.
Subjects ranging from child crime, UFOs
To Covid-19
Anything which can help stimulate the world of
Conspiracy.
Casting aspersions over Bill Gates who they
Claim has no medical history.
Stating that a cure can only make money if
People believe that they are sick.
Conspiracists firmly preach that Bill Gates
Has used his millions.
For them to trick.

Despite the current situation here in England
There's many which still follow that
Conspiracy.
Refusing to take our precious vaccine
Trying to share their views on social media.
The facts that numbers of hospitalisation and
Deaths have drastically improved.
This being due to the vaccine, they either cannot
Or they refuse to see.

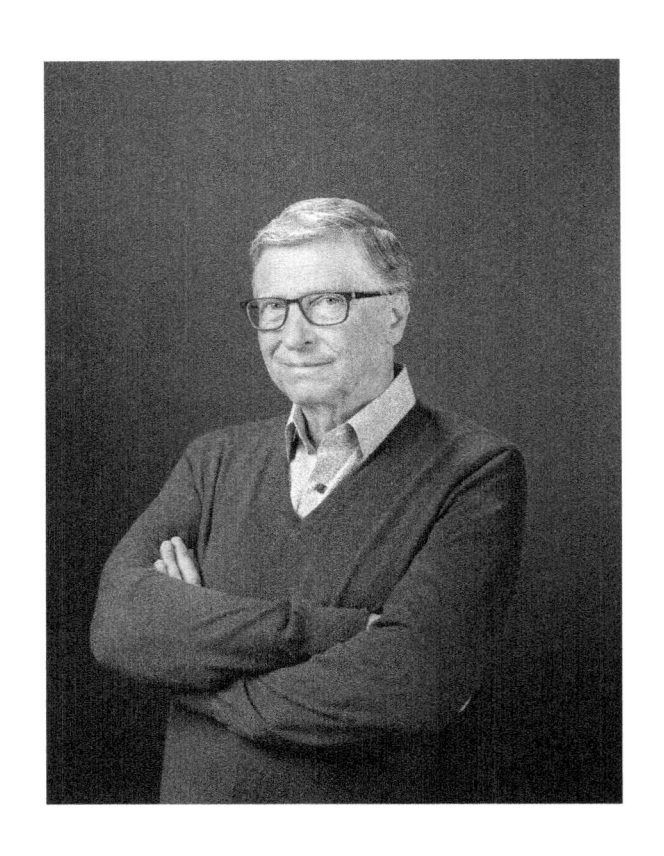

Bill Gates

Looking further around the world Its now quite
Plain to see.
That some foreign governments, on the
Vaccine rollout
They did not agree
Japan in particular is one of those
Countries who the rules it did flout
Especially in Tokyo where hospital staff are
Missing out
With our daily newspapers informing us of
Many medics in Japans hospitals
Having their hopes for a vaccine
Being left in doubt.

An oxford expert right here in England is now
Questioning the moral compass.
Of giving vaccines to our children
When world supply for adults in less rich
Countries are missing out.
As we sit and analyse the information before
Our eyes.
I am very quick to say that these government
Decisions.
On the shoulders of Boris Johnson must very
Heavily lay.

Wednesday the 19th of May in the year 2021
Downing street are briefing the
Country once again.
Matt Hancock and two medical professionals
Spoke to us from their podium
Stating that there's danger hot spots
Throughout the country
Of which Leicester is one.
This may or may not impact on opening up on
The 21st of June.

Moving forward from that Matt Hancock was
Happy to share.
About some new trials starting soon
For a booster jab to prepare.
In excess of three thousand people will now be
Required.
In order to get these vaccine trials
Up and running to the end.

Prince William this morning with the world
Has now shared.
How he has had the jab.
The Duke of Cambridge which he is known as
Attended at the Science Museum in
Kensington.
For himself and for his country a good job he
Has done.

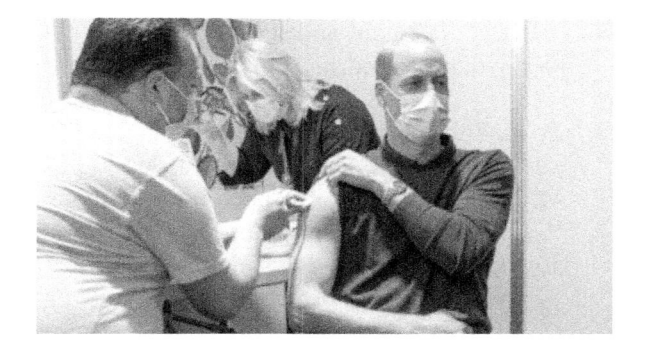

Looking at our news this morning it all feels
Very dark and gloomy.
With more revelations from our scientists.
Concerning further mutations and variants.
They are now predicting the future
Of our current vaccines.
Saying Covid will eventually beat them and
Bring us to our knees.
Unless they can produce a new variety
Which Covid symptoms it would ease.

The Telegraph newspaper is one which is
Held in high esteem.
Printing their reports of what they have
Heard and seen.
To say that this morning I was then shocked
And surprised.
To read that some people here in England
Have had their phone data analysed.
Millions of us have now been tracked, our
movements for government to see.
How and if our behaviour has changed, after
Vaccination compared to pre.

Scientists at Oxford University have agreed
They have participated in this tracking.
This will potentially cause so much damage
For the future roll out of vaccines.
Researchers on this tracking programme
Held a research contract.
Which was approved by the University of Oxford.
And declared to be done Ethically.
Being approved by an ethics committee at the University.
They declared it all to be for the better good
Of the country.

The United Kingdom together with some other Countries.
Have large groups of people who are anti Vaccine.
Making public statements such as the vaccine
Is a chip.
So, governments could track and check up on People.
That data has been anonymised before its use
For research.
Is something which the anti vax groups wont Believe.

It's now Monday morning and its May 24th 2021
Boris Johnson and his government
Have shown us once again.
How they are constantly on the lookout for
Different ways to support.
These areas of the country where Covid
Outbreaks are hitting people most
And where people need to quarantine.
Acknowledging the difficulties which people
Encounter.
When living in homes which are overcrowded.

From today going forward these areas have now
Been identified.
Our government is starting a pilot scheme
Which they hope is a good drive.
Effected families will be offered alternative
Accommodation
For a two-week period whilst they are in
Isolation.
Let's hope for all of our sakes this incentive
Will be taken up by the nation.

According to the Independent newspaper
This morning.
There's some new advice from Boris
Telling people do not travel in and out of the
Indian variant effected areas.
Of which Leicester is one.
No public announcements have been made
In relation to all of this.
However, it's been placed on the government
Website by Boris.

Meanwhile in India where people are dying in
Their thousands daily.
Hundreds of people in Karnataka broke the
Covid rules.
For the funeral of a horse which they connected
To by religion.
Now the whole village has been sealed off
No one can leave or enter for
The next ten days.
Some peoples acts of stupidity is beyond my
Comprehension.

Wednesday May 26th brings some very strong
Revelations in the news.
Dominic Cummings has spoken on live TV.
Informing the world of what he choose to
State as facts which were denigrating of
Boris Johnson.
And his handling of Covid -19.

Dominic has now shared with the world how our
Prime minister.
Did not initially believe that Covid-19 was real
He had allegedly informed people in the
House of commons.
That it was swine flu and requested that he be
Injected with Coronavirus on live TV.

In terms of our health secretary Matt Hancock
Dominic Cummings twisted the knife
Hard and deep.
Telling whoever choose to listen
How our government were calling Italy for
Covid advice.
And how Hancock of his duties should now
Be relieved.

The argument within Downing street
Continues.
With Cummings hell bent on bringing
People to their knees.
Lifting the lid of inadequacies as he did.
Has been described by a long serving
Cabinet minister.
To be like nothing which he has ever
Seen.

Whilst still in the midst of this vast world
Pandemic.
Our media brought some surprising news
Today.
Sharing how Boris Johnson our prime
Minister.
And Carrie Symonds were married
Yesterday.
Having had a small ceremony to keep in
line with Covid rules.
Boris has now shown the world that he will
Do as he choose.

Dominic Cummings has spoken once again
Regarding the reasons why he is no
Longer at number 10
Stating that people should not believe all
That which they read in the media.
The many lies that others share.
I can only feel that this man a very short
Memory he does have.
Has he forgotten his own lies to everyone
Just over twelve months ago.
When he so blatantly broke the Covid rules.

Our health secretary Matt Hancock will within
The next four weeks.
Appear in front of a parliamentary
Committee.
For allegations against him to be
Overseen.
In the interim Dominic Cummings, for
Proof he will be asked.
And be told to show the evidence of all
His accusations.
Who's telling the truth let's wait and see.

Our vaccines minister Nadhim Zahawi
Has this morning shared some
Information
Telling sky news reporter Trevor Phillips
When asked about the vaccine
Being made compulsory.
That for NHS staff our government are
Certainly.
Thinking about making the vaccine
Mandatory.
That looking at the protection of the most
Vulnerable.
Just has to be their priority.
Adding that there's already a precedent for
Surgeons to be vaccinated against
Certain diseases.

It's now Tuesday morning and it's the very 1st
Day of June.
More info in the media regarding how this
Virus its journey did begin.
Some health scientists are now saying that Sars
From the lab it did leak.
That there's now some reason to believe
That Covid did likewise but accidentally.

Looking at some Covid statistics in this
Country.
We can see that there has been some
Sustainable improvement.
Vaccine has shown that the link between
Cases, hospitalisation and deaths.
Has been well and truly broken.
Scientists who are Covid experts.
Declare the relationship can and will be
Once more awoken.
.

June the 21st this year is the day which this
Country is looking forward to.
Boris has stated that's when our lockdown
Lift will be due
Scientific experts are already advising him
That looking at data tells them.
A third wave of Covid is fairly imminent
And he should defer his opening date
Better do that than let death be people's fate.

Going back to last year and looking at how
Some other countries dealt with the
Virus.
Their strategies in the main
Were quite similar to ours.
With the exception of New Zealand who's
Prime Minister exerted
All of her powers.

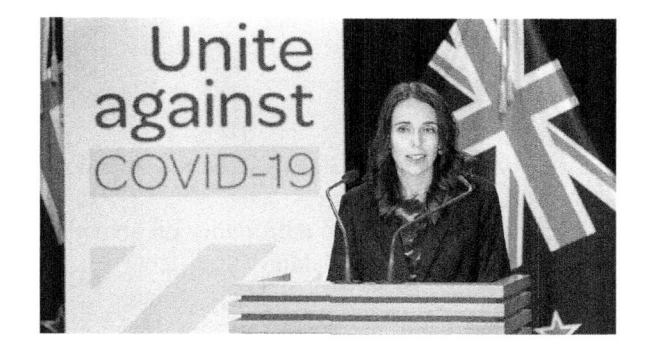

Upon hearing the news of the very 1st person
Outside of China.
Having died from Covid-19.
Jacinda Ardern took the decision which so
Many would not like.
She instantly placed restrictions on travel
Banning from her country anyone.
Coming from or via China.
Unless you were a New Zealand national
In which case for 14 days upon arrival you
Would have to self-isolate.

By early March of 2020 this lady had upped
Her game.
Everyone regardless to nationality on arrival
In New Zealand.
For fourteen days had to self-isolate.
A short time later she took a further decision.
Acknowledging that it would be the
Strictest regulation world-wide.

For the safety of her country and its people
By her rules people would have to abide.
Closing the borders to almost all non-citizens
And non-residents.
For that an apology she would avoid.

By the end of March that year her country was
In total lockdown.
The world health organisation held Jacinda in
Very high esteem.
Holding up New Zealand as an example to
So many other countries.
Stating that her fast and efficient dealing of
Covid-19.
Would have saved the lives of many.
Who without her swift action may well have
Died.

Her critics were very fast trying to cause some
Confusion.
Stating that.
With new Zealand's relatively low population.
There lay the reason for its success.
When actually it wasn't that at all but was the
Actions of its Prime minister.

Its Saturday the 5th of June with so many
Newspapers speculating.
Informing the country of a potential two
Week delay.
For all of us coming out of lockdown.
Reactions of anger to this information from
Lots of people.
Is beyond my comprehension.
Laying blame on Boris Johnson for wanting
To protect the nation.

Evidence has shown to us time and time again.
That vaccination is the only way
Out of this awful situation.
Had more people listened to our scientists in
The first instance.
Everyone over the age of thirty would now
Be vaccinated.
Meaning the ever-increasing number of
Positive tests.
Would be drastically reduced as would our
Hospital admissions.

Why are some people now blaming Boris as
This virus he did not create.
Anti Covid and anti vaxer groups.
They are rapidly spreading their hate.
Until we are officially told by our government
That we have a two-week delay.
For this country being safely able to open on
June the 21st I will pray.

Ignorance demonstrated by so many is so hard
To perceive.
All of us understanding that our economy has
Being brought to its knees.
To eventually make a full recovery is the desire
Of everyone.
That not happening any time soon
Is preferable to being shot by our own gun.

And its Sunday the 6th of June with more
Good news re the vaccine.
Pfizer and Astra Zeneca are now both
Approved.
For young people aged eleven to fifteen.
Whilst children don't especially
Get sick from Covid-19.
They can readily pass it on to others who
Are perhaps more susceptible.

Every day brings us a day closer to June the
21$^{st.}$
No decisions yet made despite the numbers
Are going up.
Our health secretary Matt Hancock in what
He says he is very clear.
It's the number of hospital admissions which
Fills him with fear.

It's now Saturday June 12th bringing decision
Day closer ever still.
People of our country surely have to now
Realise.
That we are climbing a mountain and not a
Hill.
Positive numbers from the virus.
Have more than trebled in ten days.
With the Indian variant being the problem in
Our country
From which forty-one doubly vaccinated
People have now died.

This pandemic has taken a toll in ways which
We may not consider or think about.
In India alone twenty-six thousand children
A parent they have been left without.
Reports from the international child labour
Organisation.
Makes for a very bleak read indeed.
Showing how child labour numbers are forever
Increasing.
This will not improve unless a very tight social
Protection coverage they receive.

The country has waited with baited breath
In anticipation of this day.
When Boris and his scientists to us they
Would say.
That the plan for Monday June the 21st will
Either go or stay.
Given that we watch the news the whole
Country is already aware.
That our freedom out of this lockdown
Would be too big a scare.

Boris looked so very tired a challenging job
He has to do.
Understanding all from the industry
Perspective.
We need to understand Boris too.
Speaking lots about the vaccine and how its
Saving so many lives.
For him to then want ahead of our freedom
To get more people vaccinated.
There can be no surprise.

One thing which he has now agreed from the
Previous plan
Is to let wakes and weddings go ahead with
Just one restriction when you can.
Respect the rule of social distancing with the
Number of guest's restriction no longer
Having a ban.
That's good news for many couples who have
Already so many times changed their plan.

Ignorance demonstrated by some of our fellow
Countrymen.
Still leaves me not being able to understand.
How in question time with
Boris Johnson.
Their questions felt more like a demand.
Asking him for his guarantee
That by July 19th
The whole country will be free.
How can he possibly answer that.
We will simply have to wait and see.

I'm generally speaking not a big fan of our
Prime Minister Boris Johnson.
However, throughout this pandemic he has
Worked incredibly hard.
This morning our media this country it has
Informed.
Decisions have now been finalised.
Regarding mandatory vaccination in the care
Sector.
Of which staff have been pre-warned.

A sixteen-week window is what will now be
Allowed.
Boris and his colleagues have considered the
Safety all around.
For all of the service users in their final years
Should care staff refuse the vaccine.
Further employment they will need to find
There are some who might say this ruling isn't
Very kind.
I would say it's a good plan to keep everyone
Safe
And if you don't like the heat then the kitchen
You need to leave.

Looking forward now to the day of Monday
July the 19th
The country waits with baited breath.
The vaccine versus numbers race has begun
The onus of the outcome is now
Upon everyone.
Conspiracy theories still try to dominate our
Social media platforms
Telling us we are being poisoned is about what
We are being warned.

It's now Sunday the 20th day of June and the war
It still continues
Yet looking at news reports from around the
World.
The whole thing is quite uplifting
So many people have seen sense and taken the
Vaccine.
Its sadly the refusers who will continue to create
Those bad outcomes.
Its beyond my comprehension as to why people
Its benefits they cannot see.

Here I am again and its Thursday June the 24th
Looking at world news it shows how
Moscow.
Has had quite a shift.
On the whole its population has made a very
Slow uptake.
On the Covid-19 vaccine.
Holding the belief that it was probably fake.

We are still here on Thursday the 24th of June
Our forever prying media.
Have helped bring another family to ruin
Running a storyline about our
Health secretary Mr Matt Hancock
Exposing him for conducting an extra marital
Affair.
Those reporters they are ruthless who they hurt
They do not care.

Imagine how his wife had felt as she read those
Awfully painful headlines.
Saturday June the 26th now and Matt Hancock
Has resigned
Not due to his affair.
But due to his lack of adhering to the Covid
Rules off air
Which has been confirmed by some
Photographs
Which show him in a clench with his mistress
Gina Colandelo.

Office CCTV had been watching him in early
May of this year.
Snapping pictures of him kissing a colleague
When the rules were that we all
Of each other steered clear.
What I struggle to readily understand
Is why we're hearing of this now
And not beforehand.

Its Tuesday the 29th of June in the year of
2021.
The world has woken to more awful news
Created by England's scum.
One of our government advising scientists
Has been psychically harassed.
By two thugs.
Chris Witty showed his dignity by not
Uttering a word.
Video facial content is very clear.
Surely someone decent will recognise the
Men in question
Pass their details to our police.

Digressing from the Covid story let's take a
Look at our Royal family.
Prince Charles son Harry and his brother
William.
For several months now maybe more
They've had a fallout
Which our media continues to explore.

Harry is probably the instigator by the fact
He is so outspoken.
Having married Megan Markle, they left parts
Of their lives wide open.
He talks about the cruel situation of the loss of
Their mother.
Which he and William both endured when
They were both young children.

Harry in his younger years has often been the
Rebel child.
That was his way of dealing without a mother
Which at such a young age he was
Deprived.

Blaming his mother's death on the media
By the way in which she was pursued.
He stepped back from Royalty taking his wife
Megan and their son Archie
To build a new life.
To a place where he felt they would be safe
In Santa Barbara California.

Harry and Megan

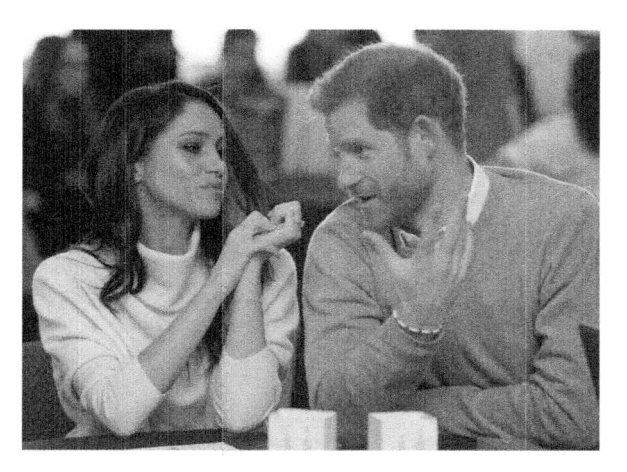

Looking at the newspapers today they highlight,
What for our school children.
Is the most awful plight
Currently throughout the United Kingdom
There's a very high quota of absenteeism.
Showing that there's three hundred and fifty-one
Thousand students away from school.
All with the Covid related rule.

We are all aware of the seriousness for us
By not sticking to the Covid rules.
This week I've spoken to someone who has
Clearly
Not done what he should do.
Telling me that his young daughter was in
Hospital with Coronavirus
But he would be at my address later on that
Afternoon
Ah no I don't think so!

Monday July the 5th and the day is dawning
Near
When we see what's happening to our rules
Regarding Covid I hope he's clear
Boris gets so many complaints from people
Who say they are confused
When he talks to the nation.

In the meantime, we have some advice from
The World Health Organisation.
An expert there has warned of easing lockdown
Restrictions too soon.
He is a respected and trustworthy gentleman
Who originates from county Mayo
More precisely Charlestown.

Looking further around the world in order to
See
What every country's doing.
New Zealand leads the way once again.
With Prime Minister Jacinda Arden and her
Colleagues in office.
Taking action to support their economy with a
20% pay cut being taken by her and them.

Jacinda Arden is a Prime Minister who takes
No messing around.
She's quick to make decisions and keeping her
Feet down on the ground.
Working with and for her people she makes
Visits to many places.
Here's a prime example of this as you can see
On the following pages.

Here on the next page is Jacinda Arden on a school visit with staff members, including my cousin Sheila White nee Flannery in the pink dress. Putting Cloontia and Ballaghaderreen on New Zealand's map. Thank you, Sheila!

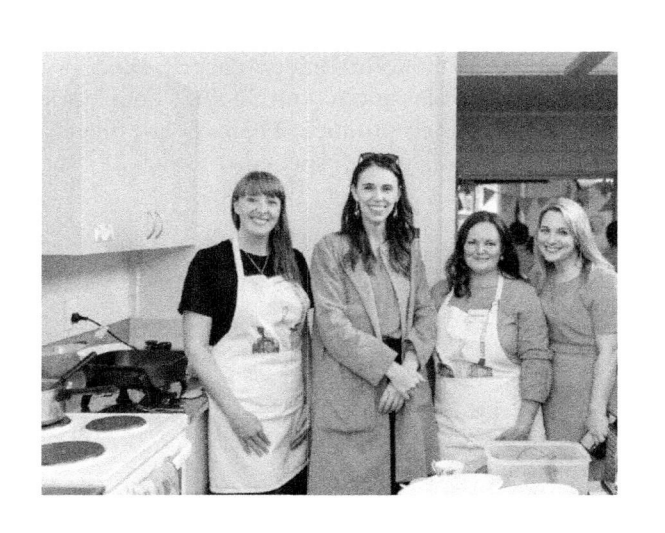

And again, on the following two pages, hand shaking in the classroom with Sheila's daughter and sampling their produce. The very last one is with the school's garden specialist Francis Clayton.

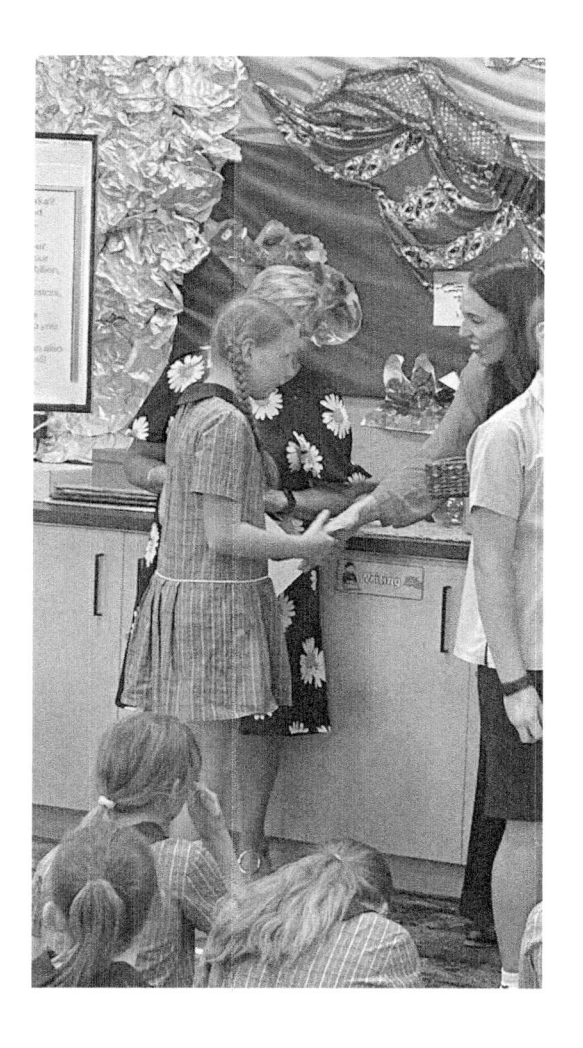

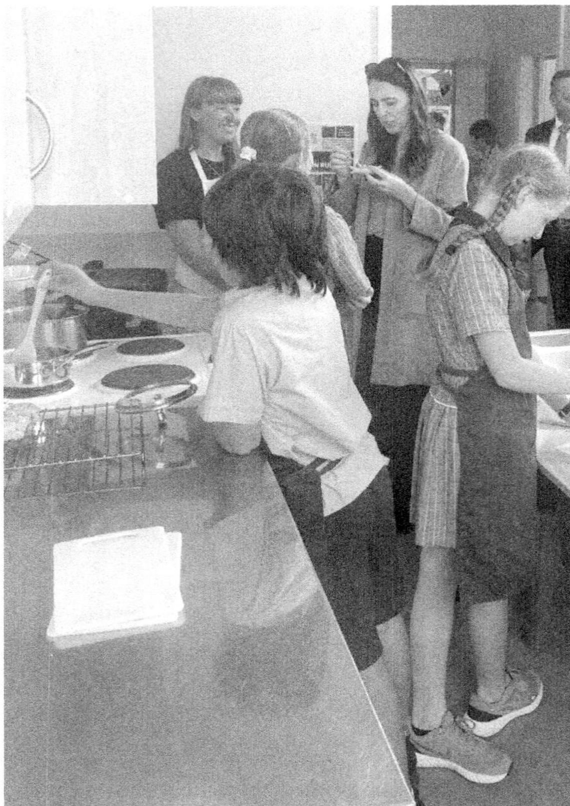

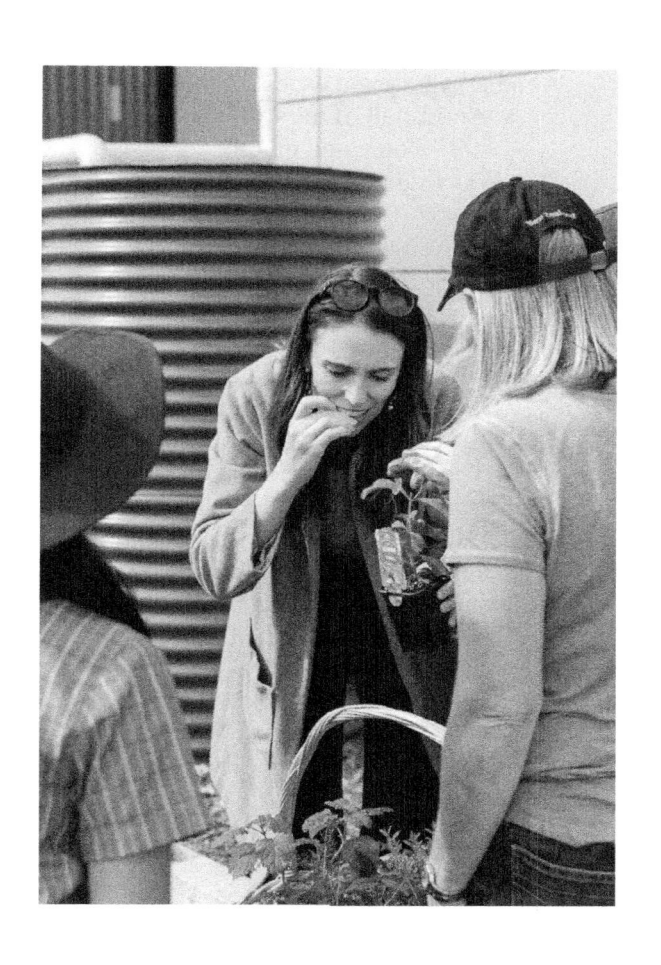

Another significant aspect of this year
Amidst all of the Covid-19
Doom and gloom.
Was England reaching the final
In the Euro 2020 football competition
Losing to Italy in a penalty shoot
Out.

Looking forward to the England games
Gave all of us so much joy
Giving a lift to the country's spirits
The lads all did us proud
Some English fans should be banned from
Our matches
As their behaviour makes me think
That had their parents used contraception
This world would be a better place
In which to live.

Everyone in this country knows that racism
Is still alive
Our penalty takers were publicly judged
By some
For the colour of their skin
Oh my god what's happened to live and let
Live.

Looking at Covid further around the world
Cases are rising drastically
Looking at our own country the same
Scenario applies
Despite this knowledge, Boris a decision he
Has made
To open up the whole country so lifting all
Of our legal restrictions
Telling the Nation to use some common
Sense.

July the 19th will be the day when everything
Will change
Returning back to almost pre Covid, is the
Man deranged?
Hundreds of doctors and scientists have now
Challenged the Prime Minister
With signatures from more than a thousand
Doctors world wide
Saying that Johnson now embarking on a herd
Immunity
Is an awful and reckless experiment.

Whilst we have had legal requirements in
Place
Thousands of people the rules they have
Disobeyed
Why then would Boris feel that its ok
To make the use of mask wearing advisory
But no longer mandatory
With the ticking of the clock leading up to
July the 19th
There's still time for a change of heart.

Meanwhile over in China for one family
There is some very good news
Back in 1997 their 2-year-old son had been
Kidnapped from outside of their house
Never giving up on the search he was in July
Of this year
Now aged 26 years
Reunited with his family by police with DNA
Proving who his parents are.

Back to Covid-19 now and its July the 16th
Three days before Boris has given
This country back its freedom.
A hospital in Birmingham has had to cancel
All operations for at least the next two days.
They have no Intensive care beds free
As all are occupied by Covid patients.

People who are waiting for their life saving
Surgery
Some of those being liver transplants whilst
Others are cancer related
This hospital has sent out warnings that this
Action in the coming weeks
May well need to be repeated
Our health service is already buckling before
The lockdown ends
Personally, I pray that ahead of Monday the 19th
That Boris might develop some common sense.

As if Covid and its variants are not enough to
Deal with.
The universe has now thrown some natural
Disasters into the mixing pot.
Currently many families in Germany
Are suffering from a broken heart.
Heavy torrential rain has brought down homes
Resulting in the death of at least.
More than 100 people
Possibly many more their lives they have lost.

World health organisation is now once again
Attempting to discover Covid-19s origin
Stating that there had been a premature push to
Rule out the theory of where it did begin
That theory being that the virus did escape
From a government lab in Wuhan
That's where the 1st human infections were
Discovered towards the end of 2019.

Doctor Tredos who is the WHO director
General, has stated that laboratory
Accidents happen.
Calling on China to be more transparent
Regarding where this virus
Its life it did begin.

As July the 19th fast approaches the world is
Looking at Boris Johnson
Wondering if he will exercise some common
Sense
Stating that his 1st line of strategy against the
Virus had ben to aim for herd immunity
Here he is now with his plan for lifting
lockdown
Reverting back to herd immunity
Once again
With 1 in every 95 people in England currently
Being Infected with Covid-19.

His plan to the world doesn't make any sense
Elsewhere around the world there's unrest
And violation
With some people from Durban making
Chaos their creation
Starting due to the jailing of an ex-president
Jacob Zuma
Creating the worst violence this area has
Seen over many years.

What is wrong with some people worldwide
Thinking this type of behaviour
Will bring many better things to their life
Zuma was jailed for his lack of appearance
..At a corruption enquiry
Days later more than two hundred people
To the violence have lost their life.

Back to home ground now with our new
Health secretary
Testing positive for Covid over the weekend
Boris and other government officials have
Been in close contact
But guess what, from self-isolating they tell
Us that they are exempt
Testing out a new pilot scheme,
They have one rule for us and a different one
For them.

Here we are again still on the same day as
Above
Boris due to much backlash now tells us that
The new pilot scheme they were testing
Has been given the shove
That just like the rest of us he and his
Colleagues will now self-isolate
Here's hoping he might also change the rules
On the imminent lockdown lifting
Before it's too late.

Now we have the 19th of July upon us our
Prime minister has refused.
To change the plans forthwith.
From this morning going forward people of
This country.
Can revert back to almost what it was like
Pre Covid-19.

From his home in isolation Boris has made the
Request.
That in terms of public busy places
That people would do their best.
With his next breath he has told the country
That if you so choose.
To a night club you may go, will people really
Wear a mask, I don't think so.
All the legal restrictions have now gone, people
Can behave more or less as they want.

Having given us yet another press conference
Boris has this evening given
The country some ultimatums
Pointing out what plans they have in mind.
Informing us that there's three million
People between the ages of
18 and 30 years
Who have been invited to take the vaccine but
Declined.

The opening up of night clubs will for almost
All young people.
Meet one of their greatest desires.
For now, they have to evidence a negative.
Test for admission
From the end of September everyone entering
Such super spreading venues.
Will require a Covid passport showing they
Have taken the vaccine.

Scientists Chris Whitty and Professor Jonathan
Van Tam
Both came out in support of what Boris
Had to say
Informing us that their expectations are
At least one thousand people being admitted
To hospital per day
Appealing to the country to do the right
Thing
Why would some people do that now when
They haven't done
From the beginning.

Waking up this morning to what feels like a
Beautiful day
There's a write up in the newspapers
By a doctor William Hanage
Who is a professor from Harvard University
In the United States.
This gentleman has stated that seeing
England's
Response to Covid-19
Has left him with feelings of profound shock.

Looking at the media this morning its quite
Frightening indeed
For the many people who to Boris
They didn't pay
Much heed
People who have recovered from Covid-19
Are not yet out of the woods
Long Covid is a real condition
Impacting the lives of many
Who have not fully recovered as they should.

Here we are almost into August and to a
Wedding I have been invited.
With gratitude I sent my acknowledgement
And acceptance.
That was many months ago, now the time is
Getting very near.
I am quite full with fear.
Of how Covid safe the venue is going to be.
And how Covid aware the guests will be.

This morning Tuesday July the 27th and the
Media has brought some good news.
Rate of Covid infections have been
Dropping.
Quite considerably over the past seven days
Boris has spoken once again, reminding the
Country to take great care.
Of his changing rules and advice
We have all had more than our fair share.

Thursday July the 29th and yet more updated
Covid news.
From November the 11th some people will be
Working under different rules
If you're a care home employee you have to
Be doubly vaccinated.
Or your job you will lose.

Many people are complaining about the above
My view is they haven't done it soon enough
People of this country who have been its
Back bone
Now need to know they're safe if ending up
In a care home.

It's now Friday the 30th of July 2021
And again, the media have
Some updated Covid news.
Showing how 99% of pregnant women
Hospitalised due to the virus
Are not vaccinated.
Through their own choice
With 1 in every 10 going to Intensive care.

Since February the 1st 2021- 742 pregnant
Women have had hospital admission
With the Coronavirus.
220 of that number were admitted just last
Week.
Those statistics have come from many
Sources.
Including Professor Marian Knight from
The University of Oxford.
Stating that there's more pregnant women
Being more severely affected
By the new Delta variant.

All of those statistics and this information
Simply goes to show
How unpredictable this awful disease can be
And despite their best of the best efforts
How little our scientists still know
Coronavirus is definitely the biggest
Challenge
This world has ever seen
Bigger than the world wars as that enemy its
Movements could be seen.

Now that the time for mandatory vaccination
For certain jobs is almost upon us.
Claims are flying around that Vegans can
Have exemption.
If I had a loved one living in a care home
I would remove them
If their staff were exempt.
I can anticipate this rule creating very many
Difficulties.
Not just for the home but for the staff
Working within it.

For the people here in England, who now feel
That maybe Boris is being unfair.
Should cast their eyes and ears towards the
Philippines
And hear what their President has to say.
Telling people who don't want the vaccine
That from his perspective they can just die
Should they leave their homes they will be
Arrested.
As their outdoor presence would make them
Walking spreaders.

It's now Sunday the very 1st day of August and
The media are at it again.
Sharing parts of an interview which they held
With Professor Adam Finn.
His expert view is that we will see Covid -19
Every year.
Into the minds of many people this will
Instil some fear.
Just like influenza Covid will still be around
I'm thinking that people will need to take
Responsibility.
And keep their feet on the ground.

Whilst we are now all living in the midst of
Covid-19
Life continues with knife crime escalating
Taking life away from so very many
Just about every day you see it on the news
Boris has made a promise to throw some more
Money at controlling it
Will he be successful is many people's views?

In Thailand many people are forgotten and
Not given the protection
Or the care which they so badly need
Buddhist monks are now donning personal
Protection gear
Then taking oxygen cylinders, taking swabs to
Help with testing
Picking up dead bodies for the crematorium
Doing all of this despite their Covid fear.

It's now Monday and the 2nd day of August
I'm looking at the media again.
Doctors and nursing staff from our hospitals
Are sharing about how it was way back then
When the virus it did begin
Talking about how they had to quarantine
Away from their families
For the family's protection
Yet the staff kept going, so much
Credit to them
In excess of 3,600 medical staff caught and
Died from Covid
In the first year alone.

Some stories they have relayed to us, on their
Minds it must prey
Of extremely sad situations
They encountered day by day.
Speaking of when people died in their beds
All alone.
Holding up Ipads with goodbye messages
And how people were too weak to pick up a
Phone.

There's some further worrying news too
A document has been leaked and exposed
Its written by the government
Scientific advisory group for emergencies
It states that a new Covid variant which is
Possibly expected
Could fight through all the vaccines
Killing people with numbers as high as
One in every three.

Other scientists supporting this document
States the above is not a possibility
But more a guarantee.
My biggest fear at this point is for my adult
Children, my grandchildren and so on
Down the line.
What an awfully cruel world in which they
Will have to live.

It's now Tuesday the 3rd day of August with
Some timely reminders
In the news
Of how New Zealand has dealt with the
Pandemic
And of the Prime Ministers views
Jacinda Arden will next week be looking at
How after sixteen long months
She can and will open up New Zealand's
Borders
From some of the toughest travel restrictions
This world has ever seen.

Back here in England our NHS now has a new
Head
What Amanda Richards has said I have read
She stated that in the past four weeks
That 20% of patients admitted to hospital with
Coronavirus
Are in the age bracket of eighteen to thirty
Four
Young people going forward for their vaccine
She would like to see more.

Its Sunday the 8th day of August and here
We are again
Reporters in the media talking about how
Covid it did begin
No one having absolute certainty on that
Scientists are now attempting to prove
Their theories
Of how this awful disease is spread.

Many continuing to say that its airborne
Whilst others disagree
With all stating that after almost two years
There's still lots of uncertainty
However, whatever the cause of its spread
Might be
A good reduction in infection numbers
This country can now see.

Monday August the 9th and world news has
Highlighted this.

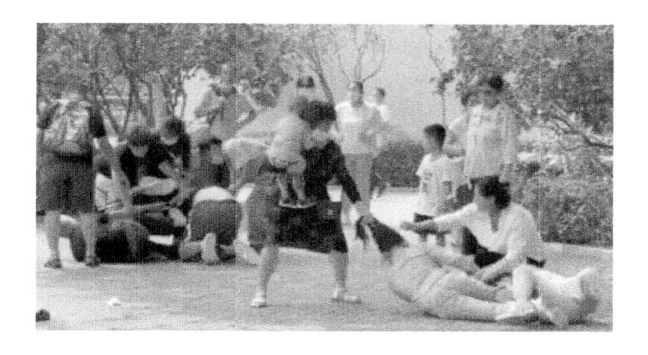

Nothing to do with Covid disgraceful as it
Is
A family over in China on a day trip
To the zoo
Having a brawl on the floor
Even the animals were in uproar
What's happened to human decency and
Respect for another
Families behaving like that in public
It's scary to think how they behave indoors
It absolutely makes me cringe seeing
That woman on the floor.

Back to the Covid story and looking at
France in particular
All visitors to the country will now have to
Prove they are doubly vaccinated
For everything including Metro travel and an
Entrance to bars, cafes and night clubs
To name but just a few
President Macron has introduced those
New rules.

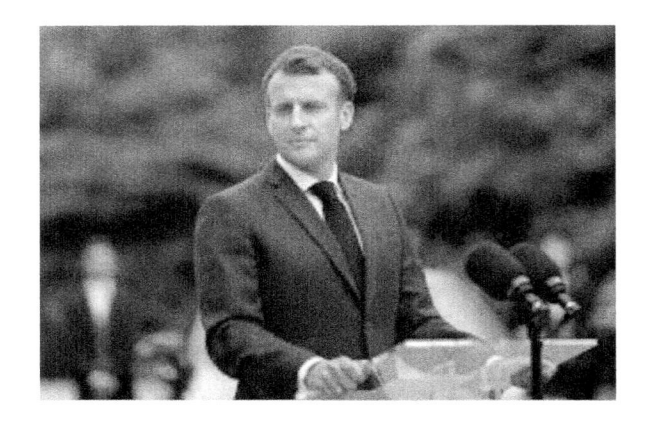

In excess of 200,000 people have taken to
The streets in protest
Many restaurant owners have stated they
Will defy the rule
Stating that such a move would kill their
Summer trade
Many have taken to social media
Stating that a red line has been crossed
By Macron bringing in those rules
To the wolves their business has been tossed.

Thursday the 12th day of August and here's
Our Coronavirus news
Jacinda Arden The New Zealand Prime
Minister
Has shared with the world what she did
Choose
Keeping her borders closed till early next
Year
Keeping Covid out she is allaying peoples
Fears.

Our country has now been opened up for
Almost 4 weeks
Getting through the expectation of numbers
Going up has been like a breeze
Whilst there has been an increase in people
Suffering from this disease
Our government is pleasantly surprised
How it's being dealt with at such ease.

Other news whilst we live with daily Covid
Updates
Brings us to our Royal family
And Prince Andrew in particular
Law suits are being brought against him by a
Female in the United States
Stating she was forced to be intimate with him
When just sixteen years of age.

Andrew is currently at Balmoral with his ex
Wife
And his mother the Queen
The palace has remained silent on
Andrews situation
How it will turn out
Remains to be seen.

It's now Monday the 16th day of August
Our media brings us some
More Covid rules
As of this morning providing you have
Been doubly vaccinated
Or you are under the age of 18 years
There's no longer a need
For close contacts of a positive to
Self-isolate.
This feels like another cautious attempt to
Bring us back to normality indeed.

Our government have taken a further step
With the rollout of the vaccine
They've made a statement that all 16-18
Year olds
Will by August the 23rd
Be offered their first vaccine
Thus giving two weeks protection
Ahead of their return to education.

With a desire to support the rollout
Many companies have stepped
Up to the mark
Offering financial incentives to
Young people, who can prove they have
Had the jab.

Meanwhile around the world and Australia
In particular
Infection rates and deaths are rising fast
Vaccinated numbers are low
Considering it's a wealthy country
You'd wonder why with the vaccine rollout
They have been so incredibly slow.

Why can't other countries take example
From New Zealand
One positive case has been found in
Auckland
It's the first in the last six months
Jacinda Arden has done as she usually does
In order to keep this contained
She has put the country back under strict
Lockdown
For 3 days in the whole of the country and 7
Days in Auckland
This is a community infection with no links
To the borders.

The Taliban have now once again invaded
Afghanistan
To the detriment of especially Afghan
Ladies and girls
People are scrambling in their hundreds
To leave the country
Ahead of the oppression they will suffer
If they don't.

Boris Johnson has made a promise that he
Will allow some over here
It's a humanitarian action to take
How that will impact our Covid situation
I'm guessing it will be negative.

Meanwhile New Zealand has spoken once
Again
To the country and to the world
Going to extraordinary lengths to prevent
Outbreaks
With an amazing contact trace response
To its one single case.

The three-day lockdown initially imposed has
Now been extended to seven
Government have identified every place the
Stricken man has been
Public have been informed and told that if they
Too were in those places they now need to
Self-isolate
What a lady Jacinda Arden is.

Lots of debate going on in parliament
In relation to the booster vaccine
Scientists and government chopping and
Changing their minds
Re who should get it
And their reasons why.

Last night in London saw a huge surge of
People
Storm our ITN studios I think they are almost
Evil
Shouting out their protests against the
Vaccine
I believe they're just trouble makers
Who on television they want to be seen.

As if Covid infection is not enough for the
World to deal with right now
Human rights for people in Afghanistan
Are rapidly disappearing
The Taliban having taken control once
More
With people scrambling in the thousands
To leave its shore.

Some have now already died from being
Trampled at the airport
In attempts to leave before August the 31st
From that day the Taliban have said
Kabul airport will be closed with no one
Ever allowed to leave again.

Afghan people and all others in the country
Will now live under Taliban rule
Where women are badly disrespected
Having their human rights removed.
Where gay people will be tracked down and
Killed.

The Taliban say that to be gay is punishable
By death under Sharia law
Having already beaten a gay man to death
Then chopped his body into pieces
No one in this world should have to live
With such fear.

Kabul airport is now largely destroyed by a
Suicide bomber
Which also took the lives of very many
Innocent people
Our foreign secretary Mr Dominic Raab
Had allegedly been informed
Of the Taliban potential takeover
Several weeks before it occurred.

It's now Friday August the 3rd 2021
How some parts of the world are
Dealing with Covid
Really is not much fun
Having family in Idaho I'm feeling very
Scared indeed
Out there the vaccine has not really been
Shared
People filling up the hospitals in their
Intubated beds
That's more to do with people's refusal than
A vaccine stock supply.

Closer to home now our numbers continue to
Rise
Schools are back so there's more infection
We need to keep open our eyes
Our scientists have eventually passed the
Pfizer
For anyone aged over sixteen
My two granddaughters have now been
Vaccinated
I'm hoping that for my grandsons both aged
Fourteen
The red light will soon go ahead.

Meanwhile throughout the country there are
Protestors galore
Including where I took my granddaughter
For her vaccine
People there were on the floor
Brandishing their placards
Saying stop killing your child
Police presence helped keep everyone in
Line.

Whilst the world grapples with Covid there's
Been the most unthinkable accident
Elsewhere
Twin boys aged twenty months have had an
Experience
Beyond the realms of being unfair
It's said that a parent had driven them to
Their day-care
Then forgot they were in the car
That occurred in South Carolina on
Wednesday of this week
Parent returned to their car nine hours later
To find both boys from heat stroke
They were now deceased.

Back in New Zealand numbers have now
Risen
Despicable behaviour has been exhibited
By one man in particular
Attempting three times to remove himself
From his place of isolation
On the fourth attempt he was successful
With zero regard for the nation.

His mother did an action which would have
Been incredibly hard to do
She called the local law enforcers
Who found and returned him back to the
Venue
He now has an armed guard outside
Of his bedroom door
Until his isolation period has been completed
And he is a risk no more.

Here we are now on the 6th day of September
There has previously been some talk of
Covid passports
As we all remember
Our health secretary together with the prime
Minister
Have informed the media that this will come
To pass
By the end of September.

It's now Monday morning the 13th of September
Our media brings the country some more
Covid news
Boris Johnson has once again done a U
Turn
Regarding Covid passports and their use.

Previous government guidelines had stated
That to enter a night club or other
Potentially busy venue
That from September People would
Need to show their
Vaccination passport and now
The rule is that they don't.
Media this morning brings us further news

The artist Nicki Minaj has been
Sharing her Covid views
Stating how she did not attend the Met Gala
Awards evening
She is spreading rumours of never spoken
About side effects.

Not being vaccinated herself she says she is
Doing research and
That a family member after vaccination has
Become impotent
Nowhere in the world has that side effect
Been listed
Nicki Minaj it appears is quite anti vaccine.

Looking at all around the world we can
Surely see
How everywhere we look and listen
There are people who will be
Pushing their own agenda
In attempts to make people stop
And refuse the vaccine.

Some other news to take our attention away
From the virus
We all know know how our country has
Deteriorated
I'm referring here to gun and knife crime
So many have lost their lives at the hands
Of that brutality
Get arrested, go to go court walk away with
An order to do work in the community.

Down in Whitechapel last Sunday in the very
Early evening
A new type of behaviour returned to our
Streets
People have had enough, now the new way
Of
Dealing out punishments has begun.
A perpetrator of those crimes who has been
Going to certain areas instilling fear.
Has been attacked by a group of vigilantes
Being relieved of his machette by them.

The young man then had instilled into him some
Fear.
They simply chopped off his hand from the
Wrist
With the machette he was using to torture
Others
Then walked away with the machette leaving
Him with hand on ground in a pool of
Blood.

Whilst people generally speaking may not
Believe
That being a vigilante is the right thing to do
If this allows the decent people who have
Been failed by the courts, to go out
Without fear and be safe
Then it's definitely all right by me and I hope
By you too.

Hopefully this man losing his hand and in
Such a gruesome way too
May serve as a lesson to others contemplating
Instilling fear, torture and murder.
As now the vigilantes have started in this
Gruesome manner
They are going to continue and will hopefully
Make our country a much safer place to be.

Back now to the Covid story on Friday the 17th
Of September.
Italy is now leading the world with its new
Restrictions.
Covid green pass will be required for every
Employee.
On October 15th this will become
Mandatory.

Failure of compliance to the rule will bring
Penalties which are severe.
Job suspension with loss of pay
It may also mean a hefty fine.
The sole purpose behind this new green pass
Is to keep people safe.
And increase the volume of vaccinations
Administered along the way.

Now Saturday the 18th of September the
Media reports of a leak of government
Information.
Stating that whilst Boris on Tuesday
September the 14th had told our
Country.
That he has two Covid plans for over
Winter here in England.

Plan A would be for everyone to take the
Advice to wear a mask.
To social distance when you can
Unvaccinated should take up their offer
Those who are offered it should take the
Booster vaccine.

Plan B would be potentially that the most
Strict and severe plans
Would be the reintroduction of the
Wearing of masks mandatory
Together with a Covid vaccine pass for our
Entry to public indoor space.

Boris stated very clearly that plans A and B
Are and have to be the only way forward
For our country
When asked about further lockdowns
Should our numbers escalate further more
Boris denied there was any thought or any
Consideration of a plan C.

Our environment minister can be heard in
An interview
Stating that yes there is a plan C
George Eustice in that interview
He did concede.
That government have considered the option of
Another full lockdown for our country
Should there be a new variant which resists
The vaccine
Why oh why does Boris have to lie?

Sunday the 19th of September in the year of 2021
Media inform us that the deals are now done
Previous prime minister Mr Tony Blair
Has advised Boris Johnson
That's a scenario which is quite rare
Stating to the government that Boris should
Skip plan A
That now is the time to go direct to plan B
Will Boris be advised we will see.

It's now Tuesday the 21st of September 2021
Worldwide news and media are showing
Us once again.
How the vaccination uptake in Florida has
Really slowed down a great deal.
Right-wing talk radio presenters in the state
Are considered to be the driving force
With programme presenters who are
Anti-vaccine.
Five of those anti-vax presenters have lost
Their lives to Covid
Over the past few weeks.

The worlds becoming crazier than it ever has
Done before
In Melbourne in Australia people are in
Absolute uproar
Violent anti-vax protestors
Have taken to the streets
Police officers on horseback have been
Brought to their knees.

It's now Wednesday September the 22nd
And the Covid story will continue
From China comes a new revelation
This appears to be a legitimate document
Leaked proposals show that from 2018
Scientists in China had a plan to release
Enhanced Coronavirus
Into the Chinese bat population to inoculate
Them against the disease which could
Jump to humans
Funding for their programme was declined.

It's Sunday the 26th of September and looking at
World Covid news
The manager of a funeral home in Idaho
Namely Mr Salove
Has shared with the Washington news
How his morgue is over full due to deaths
From the Corona Virus
Other funeral homes are near tipping point too.

Mr Salove this week has made the decision to
Provide a refrigerated trailer
To take extra capacity over and above
The usual number of bodies which
Can be accommodated
And to hold the growing number of the dead
Oh lord why don't people become
Vaccinated.

Almost the end of the month of September
We now have many shortages here in
England
Ranging from supermarket shelves being
Empty
To ques over a mile long at some petrol
Stations.

Those problems have arisen due to our
Brexit rules
The removal of foreign drivers' visas
Has created a shortage of lorry drivers too
Now Boris is doing a turn around
Stating that visas can be reinstated until
Towards the end of December
What is the man thinking?
European drivers return to their country
Our shortage problems will remain.

Friday the 1st day of October in the year of 2021
Once again, our media brings us some news
Regarding virus immunity for some.
Scientists who have done deep research
Have discovered this news to be true.

Stating that people who have had Covid and
Recovered, and then given the vaccine
They have antibodies which are capable of
Neutralising the two variants we have so far
Seen
Plus, neutralising viruses which are much
More diverse.

Thursday the 21st day of October in the year
Of 2021
The fear of yet a further lockdown
For England has now begun
Covid infection cases are soaring very high
Many people are going to hospital
With a fear that they will probably need to
Go to intensive care or maybe
They will die.

Friday the 22nd day of October and here we
Are again
An anti-vaxer man walked in to Colchester
Hospital
Surrounded by a small group of other men
Handing some fake legal documents
To a member of the NHS
With an accusation of them committing
Crimes against humanity
Stating that Covid is a hoax and they are
Operating illegally.

Personally, I now am fully vaccinated
Having had my booster jab
Last week
However, I am not complacent
Around the Covid rules
I will always them obey.

Monday the 15th day of November in the
Year of 2021
Today we had some more news
From professor Van Dan Tamme
Emphasis being on the vaccine uptake
Stating how the booster should give some
lengthy immunity.

Meantime lots of care home staff who have
Remained antivax
Have now after warning
Been given the sack
Some are seen leaving in tears
My thoughts are with Boris, eliminating
Residents and their families fears.

Thursday the 18th day of November 2021
And here we are again
Governments of two European countries
Are putting people's heads in a spin
Enforcing lockdown of the unvaccinated
Just how is that going to be policed
I'm guessing it will be Covid passport
Where ever people attempt to meet.

Meanwhile back here in England our data
Shows
Numbers of transmission have increased
As per usual Boris Johnson is doing little
Other than telling the nation the storm clouds
Are gathering in Europe
Will he be forced to implement our plan B
Yes, we all remember what happened when
The waves started rolling in
The question is does he?

Thursday the 25th day of November 2021
Media brings some more tragic news
Regarding a young Scottish woman
Who has just died from the virus
Her father has spoken to the media
Sending out a special appeal
Saying that if his daughter had been
Vaccinated
She would still be here.

Very very tragic circumstances have hit
This family hard
Leaving three young children behind her
From a situation which people can avoid
Her father is so very angry from
Their obvious devastation.
He has called on Boris Johnson
To send out a message to the nation.

Telling people to get the vaccine or else
They get a hefty fine.
Making the whole thing mandatory
The country would soon get in line
His daughter was not an anti vaxer
She simply didn't make the time.

Saturday November the 27th and more news
To be shared
There's a new variant of Corona virus
Mutated in some African countries
Boris has put travel restrictions on five of
Those countries
Where travel is not allowed to the United
Kingdom
Unless your Irish or British returning back
Home.

For people who may return from those five
Countries.
They are faced with a very heavy expense
Having to go to a government chosen hotel
For a period of ten days isolation.
Those countries now being on the red list for
Travel to the United Kingdom
Sounds as though that's offering us some
Protection
From this highly transmissible and infectious
Covid variant.
My own thoughts are will it ever end?

Meanwhile as we do battle with Covid-19
And all which that entails
Awful things are happening in this world
Which leaves you biting at your nails
People smuggling groups are offering
Small boats and dinghy's too
People from faraway lands are crossing the
Channel in those dinghy's as they do.

Most recently last week one such boat was
On its way from France
Overloaded with migrants on their way to
The UK
High winds and poor conditions combined
With low quality and an unsafe
Dinghy
Caused the Dinghy to capsize
Resulting in the loss of at least 27 lives
So awfully sad.

Back here in England crime seems to be
Out of control
Almost every day our media brings to us
News of murders untold
Generally, its women being murdered by
Men
The youngest this week being a 12-year-old
Girl in Liverpool
Who through an argument was set upon and
Murdered by 3 young men.

Many people as do I feel the courts do not
Give strong enough deterrents
I'm wondering if it's now time to bring back
The death penalty
Thus, allowing people to live in a country
With less fear when they go outside
I personally am full of fear and
Would not even take a bus ride.

Saturday November the 27th and we've
Been spoken to again
This time it was from Downing street by
Boris and his scientific men
Some old restrictions are being returned
For the good of all mankind
To wear a face mask in shops and on
Public transport is now mandatory
As two cases of this new and dangerous
Variant
In this country they did find.

Wednesday the 1st day of December 2021
Some new Covid rules have now begun
Boris has annoyed his colleagues
Saying his isolation rule is like a pun
Double vaccinated and with booster
But feeling fully well
If in contact with a positive you have to
Isolate as well
Some ministers say this is the road to hell
Boris initially said to review in 3 weeks
Now he's saying its legal for 3 months.

More news on how the new Covid strain is
Causing some world-wide concern.
The virus is still with us its thriving well and
Strong as its remaining firm
There's so much uncertainty in the world at
This time
Travel restrictions which had been lifted are
Now back in line.

World health organisation are being clear that
The vaccine is not a charitable asset.
African countries have a very low incidence
Of the vaccine.
Its less than 7 per cent.
In Botswana there are 19 confirmed cases of
The new variant.
Countries are now refusing people unless
They're double vaccinated.
Greece is making the vaccine mandatory for
Everyone over the age of 60 years.
Continued refusal of compliance will for them
Carry a fine of 100 euros per month each.

Boris has considered the reintroduction of
The rule of dining outdoors only
With consideration also given to placing
Restriction
On the meeting of people indoors in private
Homes
France has shut its borders to all to and from
The UK
This has totally ruined my son's family plans
For their Christmas day.

Boris has now stated very clearly indeed
That there will be no further restrictions
This side of Christmas day
Telling the nation to be cautious what they do
Then hopefully that's how the rule will stay
It's now looking to me that this virus will
Extend itself
Into at least one more year
For my recollections of its events from the
Very beginning
I am now going to leave it here.

Meanwhile our television on channel ITV
A blunder they did make
Speaking about Pope Francis
His death the reporter did announce
By mistake
Quickly retracting her statement
Embarrassment was evident on her face.

Here we are now in January of the year 2022
My son has got Covid as does
My grandson too.
Fortunately for them both they are vaccinated.
Illness was mild with a speedy recovery.

Our Covid situation now in February 2022
Is Boris once again changing the rules
Every legal Covid requirement
Is now coming to an end.
Four weeks ahead of that which was originally
Planned.

I'm going to wrap this up now with the
Exception of just a few.
There will be no more Covid tales from me
But this I will say.
Our government are a laughing stock
As Boris has been found out.
To have been attending parties at
Downing street.
When the rest of us were not allowed out.

The country's now waiting for the police
Investigation.
Also waiting for Boris to hand in his
Resignation.
Families lost their loved ones where and
When they died alone
As Boris and his cronies
Partied in his Downing street home
And certainly not on their own.

And finally, before I close on the 2nd of April
2022.
Despite having taken every care and caution
I myself have joined the Covid.
Chosen.
Experiencing the most severe of flu symptoms
I truly felt like I was going to die.
Those two red lines which show that we are
Covid positive.
Are still there on day 9.
Having spoken to my doctor yet again.
I now have some equivalent of penicillin.
I do like to take Captain Toms attitude.
With the expression of Tomorrows, a new day.

This memoir of those two years has been written accurately, from information heard from the television updates and read in some newspapers. I'm hoping it has given people a laugh along the way.
Other serious world matters occurring at this time- Russia has now attacked The Ukraine with the loss of very many lives. My hope is that Putin will be removed somehow- in which ever manner necessary from power.

About the author

Beatrice Finn was born and raised in a small village called Derrinabroock, in the townland of Cloontia, in County Mayo West Ireland. That was a lifetime ago in the year 1949. She lived there for the first 14 years of her life. Living with her farming parents in rural Ireland and off the grid, gave her many experiences you would not find in the classroom. Starting school at the age of 7 years, Beatrice had enjoyed a basic education. Her broader education came from the experience of living on the farm, up to the point of emigration to England. That event occurred on September 6th 1963.

Beatrice has extended her education within her career as a support worker, for the National Health Service.

Beatrice has been working for her local authority for the past 22 years. Fostering challenging teenagers is something which has enriched her life in many ways.

Printed in Great Britain
by Amazon